By the Same Author

THE NATURE OF MAN

Studies in Optimistic Philosophy. By ÉLIE METCHNIKOFF, Professor at the Pasteur Institute. The English Translation edited by P. CHALMERS MITCHELL, M.A., D. Sc. Oxon., Secretary of the Zoölogical Society of London. *Illustrated. 8º. net $2.00*

The Lancet. "Those who read this remarkable book can convince themselves that his story and the message of hope which it conveys are not the vain imaginations, but the logical inferences to be drawn from observed facts. The argument which Professor Metchnikoff unfolds in a story more fascinating than the "Arabian Nights" is that human misery and suffering are due to disturbances in our organic equilibrium which strike discords within our mortal frame and rack our flesh with the torments of Procrustes. Dr. Mitchell is not only to be congratulated on his courage in translating this volume, but also on the elegance and the refinement of the language by which he has enabled Professor Metchnikoff to present his philosophic conceptions to the English-speaking peoples."

IMMUNITY IN INFECTIVE DISEASES

By ÉLIE METCHNIKOFF, Foreign Member of the Royal Society of London, Professor at the Pasteur Institute, Paris. Translated from the French by Francis G. Binnie, of the Pathological Department, University of Cambridge. With Forty-five Figures in the Text.

Royal 8vo., pp. xvi.+592. Price $5.25 net.

Athenæum.—"The subject with which this admirable volume deals is one which has in recent years attracted a vast amount of attention, not only on account of its practical importance in medicine, but also because of the fascinating interest of the problems involved. . . . The present translation of Prof. Metchnikoff's work has been admirably carried out. . . . We have here the record of five-and-twenty years of thoughtful speculation tested by laborious experiment, and no more important book on the subject has ever appeared in the English language."

G. P. PUTNAM'S SONS

NEW YORK   LONDON

THE PROLONGATION OF LIFE

OPTIMISTIC STUDIES

BY

ÉLIE METCHNIKOFF

SUB-DIRECTOR OF THE PASTEUR INSTITUTE, PARIS

THE ENGLISH TRANSLATION

EDITED BY

P. CHALMERS MITCHELL

M.A., D.Sc. Oxon., Hon. LL.D., F.R.S.

Secretary of the Zoological Society of London; Corresponding Member of the Academy of Natural Sciences of Philadelphia

G. P. PUTNAM'S SONS
NEW YORK & LONDON
The Knickerbocker Press
1908

Printing Statement:

Due to the very old age and scarcity of this book, many of the pages may be hard to read due to the blurring of the original text, possible missing pages, missing text and other issues beyond our control.

Because this is such an important and rare work, we believe it is best to reproduce this book regardless of its original condition.

Thank you for your understanding.

EDITOR'S INTRODUCTION

ÉLIE METCHNIKOFF has carried on the high purpose of the Pasteur Institute by devoting his genius for biological inquiry to the service of man. Some years ago, in a series of Essays which were intended to be provocative and educational, rather than expository, he described the direction towards which he was pressing. I had the privilege of introducing these Essays to English readers under the title *The Nature of Man*, a Study in Optimistic Philosophy. In that volume, Professor Metchnikoff recounted how sentient man, regarding his lot in the world, had found it evil. Philosophy and literature, religion and folk-lore, in ancient and modern times have been deeply tinged with pessimism. The source of these gloomy views lies in the nature of man itself. Man has inherited a constitution from remote animal ancestors, and every part of his structure, physical, mental and emotional, is a complex legacy of diverse elements. Possibly at one time each quality had its purpose as an adaptation to environment, but, as man, in the course of his evolution, and the environment itself have changed, the old harmonious intercourse between quality and circumstances has been dislocated in many cases. And so there have come into existence many instances of what the Professor calls "disharmony," persistences of structures, or habits, or desires that are no longer useful, but even harmful, failures of parallelism between the growth, maturity and decay of physical and mental qualities and so forth. Religions and philosophies alike have failed to find remedies or efficient anodynes for these evils of existence, and, so far, man is justified of his historical and actual pessimism.

Metchnikoff, however, was able to proclaim himself an optimist, and found, in biological science, for the present generation a hope, or, at the least, an end towards which to work, and for future generations a possible achievement of that hope. Three chief evils that hang over us are disease, old age, and death. Modern science has already made vast strides towards the destruction of disease, and no one has more right to be listened to than a leader of the Pasteur Institute when he asserts his confidence that rational hygiene and preventive measures will ultimately rid mankind of disease. The scientific investigation of old age shows that senility is nearly always precocious and that its disabilities and miseries are for the most part due to preventable causes. Metchnikoff showed years ago that there exists in the human body a number of cells known generally as phagocytes, the chief function of which is to devour intruding microbes. But these guardians of the body may turn into its deadly enemies by destroying and replacing the higher elements, the specific cells of the different tissues. The physical mechanism of senility appears to be in large measure the result of this process. Certain substances, notably the poisons of such diseases as syphilis and the products of intestinal putrefaction, stimulate the activity of the phagocytes and so encourage their encroachment on the higher tissues. The first business of science is to remove these handicaps in favour of the wandering, corroding phagocytes. Specific poisons must be dealt with

EDITOR'S INTRODUCTION

separately, by prevention or treatment, and it is well known that Metchnikoff has made great advances in that direction. The most striking practical side of *The Nature of Man*, however, was the discussion of the cause and prevention of intestinal putrefaction. Metchnikoff believes that the inherited structure of the human large intestine and the customary diet of civilised man are specially favourable to the multiplication of a large number of microbes that cause putrefaction. The avoidance of alcohol and the rigid exclusion from diet of foods that favour putrefaction, such as rich meats, and of raw or badly cooked substances containing microbes, do much to remedy the evils. But the special introduction of the microbes which cause lactic fermentation has the effect of inhibiting putrefaction. By such measures Metchnikoff believes that life will be greatly prolonged and that the chief evils of senility will be avoided. It may take many generations before the final result is attained, but, in the meantime, great amelioration is possible. There remains the last enemy, death. Metchnikoff shows that in the vast majority of cases death is not "natural," but comes from accidental and preventable causes. When diseases have been suppressed and the course of life regulated by scientific hygiene, it is probable that death would come only at an extreme old age. Metchnikoff thinks that there is evidence enough at least to suggest that when death comes in its natural place at the end of the normal cycle of life, it would be robbed of its terrors and be accepted as gratefully as any other part of the cycle of life. He thinks, in fact, that the instinct of life would be replaced by an instinct of death.

Metchnikoff's suggestion, then, was that science should be encouraged and helped in every possible way in its task of removing the diseases and habits that now prevent human life from running its normal course, and his belief is that were the task accomplished, the great causes of pessimism would disappear.

In this new volume, *The Prolongation of Life*, the main thesis is carried further, and a number of criticisms and objections are met. The latter, so far as they relate to technical details, I need say nothing of here, as Metchnikoff and his staff at the Pasteur Institute are the most skilled existing technical experts on these matters, but I cannot refrain from a word of comment on the brilliant treatment of the objection to the suggested amelioration of human life that it considered only the individual and neglected the just subordination of the individual to society. In the sixth Part of this volume, Metchnikoff discusses the relation of the individual to the species, society or colony, from the general point of view of comparative biology, and shows that as organisation progresses, the integrity of the individual becomes increasingly important. Were orthobiosis, the normal cycle of life, attained by human beings, there still would be room for specialisation of individuals and for differentiation of the functions of individuals in society, but instead of the specialisation and differentiation making individuals incomplete throughout their whole lives, they would be distributed over the different periods of the life of each individual.

As these lines are intended to be an introduction, not a commentary, I will now leave the reader to follow the argument in the book itself.

P. CHALMERS MITCHELL.

LONDON, *August*, 1907.

PREFACE

It is now four years since I wrote a volume, the English translation of which was called *The Nature of Man,* and which was an attempt to frame an optimistic conception of life. Human nature contains many very complex elements, due to its animal ancestry, and amongst these there are some disharmonies to which our misfortunes are due, but also elements which afford the promise of a happier human life.

My views have encountered many objections, and I wish to reply to some of these by developing my arguments. This was my first task in this book, but I have also brought together a series of studies on problems which closely affect my theory.

Although it has been possible to support my conception by new facts, some of which have been established by my fellow-workers, others by myself, there still remain many sides of the subject where it is necessary to fall back on hypotheses. I have accepted such imperfections instead of delaying the publication of my book.

Even at present there are critics who regard me as incapable of sane and logical reasoning. The longer I postpone publication, the longer would I leave the field open to such persons. What I have been saying may serve also as a reply to the remark of one of my critics, that my ideas have been "suggested by self-preoccupation."

It is, of course, quite natural that a biologist whose attention had been aroused by noticing in his own case the phenomena of precocious old age should turn to study the causes of it. But it is equally plain that such a study could give no hope of resisting the decay of an organism which had already for many years been growing old. If the ideas which have come out of my work bring about some modification in the onset of old age, the advantage can be gained only by those who are still young, and who will be at the pains to follow the new knowledge. This volume, in fact, like my earlier one on the "Nature of Man," is directed much more to the new generation than to that which has already been subjected to the influence of the factors which produce precocious old age. I think that thus the experience of those who have lived and worked for long can be made of service to others.

As this volume is a sequel to *The Nature of Man*, I have tried as much as possible to avoid repetition of what was fully explained in the earlier volume.

Here I bring together the results of work that has been done since the publication of *The Nature of Man*. Some of the chapters relate to subjects upon which I have lectured, or which, in a different form, have been printed before. For instance, the section on the psychic rudiments of man appeared in the *Bulletin de l'Institut général psychologique* of 1904, the essay on Animal Societies was published in the *Revue Philomatique de Bordeaux et du Sud-Ouest* of 1904, and in the *Revue* of J. Finot of the same year, whilst a German translation of it appeared in Prof. Ostwald's *Annalen der Naturphilosophie*. The chapter on soured milk first appeared as a pamphlet, published in

PREFACE

1905. The substance of my views on natural death was published in June last in "Harper's Monthly Magazine" of New York, while the chapter on natural death in animals appeared in the first number of the *Revue du Mois* for 1906.

I have to thank most sincerely the friends and pupils who have helped me by bringing before me new facts, or other materials; the names of these will appear in their proper places in the volume. I have not mentioned by name, however, Dr. J. Goldschmidt, whose continual encouragement and practical sympathy have made my work much easier.

Finally, my special thanks are due to Drs. Em. Roux and Burnet, and M. Mesnil, who have been so good as to correct my manuscript and the proofs of this volume.

É. M.

PARIS, *Feb.* 7, 1907.

CONTENTS

	PAGE
EDITOR'S INTRODUCTION	v
PREFACE	ix

PART I

THE INVESTIGATION OF OLD AGE

I

THE PROBLEMS OF SENILITY

Treatment of old people in uncivilised countries.—Assassination of old people in civilised countries.—Suicide of old people.—Public assistance in old age.—Centenarians.—Mme. Robineau, a lady of 106 years of age.—Principal characters of old age.—Examples of old mammals.—Old birds and tortoises.—Hypothesis of senile degeneration in the lower animals 1

II

THEORIES OF THE CAUSATION OF SENILITY

Hypothesis of the causation of senility.—Senility cannot be attributed to the cessation of the power of reproduction of the cells of the body.—Growth of the hair and the nails in old age.—Inner mechanism of the senescence of the tissues.—Notwithstanding the criticisms of M. Marinesco, the neuronophags are true phagocytes.—The whitening of hair, and the destruction of nerve cells as arguments against a theory of old age based on the failure of the reproductive powers of the cells 15

III

MECHANISM OF SENILITY

Action of the macrophags in destroying the higher cells.—Senile degeneration of the muscular fibres.—Atrophy of the skeleton.—Atheroma and arterial sclerosis.—Theory that Old Age is due to alteration in the vascular glands.—Organic tissues that resist phagocytosis 25

PART II
LONGEVITY IN THE ANIMAL KINGDOM

I
THEORIES OF LONGEVITY

Relation between longevity and size.—Longevity and the period of growth.—Longevity and the doubling in weight after birth.—Longevity and rate of reproduction.—Probable relations between longevity and the nature of the food . . 39

II
LONGEVITY IN THE ANIMAL KINGDOM

Longevity in the lower animals.—Instances of long life in sea-anemones and other vertebrates.—Duration of life of insects.—Duration of life of "cold-blooded" vertebrates.—Duration of life of birds.—Duration of life of mammals.—Inequality of the duration of life in males and females.—Relations between longevity and fertility of the organism . 47

III
THE DIGESTIVE SYSTEM AND SENILITY

Relations between longevity and the structure of the digestive system.—The cæca in birds.—The large intestine of mammals.—Function of the large intestine.—The intestinal microbes and their agency in producing auto-intoxication and auto-infection in the organism.—Passage of microbes through the intestinal wall 59

IV
MICROBES AS THE CAUSE OF SENILITY

Relations between longevity and the intestinal flora.—Ruminants.—The horse.—Intestinal flora of birds.—Intestinal flora of cursorial birds.—Duration of life in cursorial birds.—Flying mammals.—Intestinal flora and longevity of bats.—Some exceptions to the rule.—Resistance of the lower vertebrates to certain intestinal microbes . . . 73

CONTENTS

V
DURATION OF HUMAN LIFE

Longevity of man.—Theory of Ebstein on the normal duration of human life.—Instances of human longevity.—Circumstances which may explain the long duration of human life 84

PART III
INVESTIGATIONS ON NATURAL DEATH

I
NATURAL DEATH AMONGST PLANTS

Theory of the immortality of unicellular organisms.—Examples of very old trees.—Examples of short-lived plants.—Prolongation of the life of some plants.—Theory of the natural death of plants by exhaustion.—Death of plants from auto-intoxication 94

II
NATURAL DEATH IN THE ANIMAL WORLD

Different origins of death in animals.—Examples of natural death associated with violent acts.—Examples of natural death in animals without digestive organs.—Natural death in the two sexes.—Hypothesis as to the cause of natural death in animals 109

III
NATURAL DEATH AMONGST HUMAN BEINGS

Natural death in the aged.—Analogy of natural death and sleep.—Theories of sleep.—*Ponogenes.*—The instinct of sleep.—The instinct of natural death.—Replies to critics.—Agreeable sensation at the approach of death . . . 119

PART IV
SHOULD WE TRY TO PROLONG HUMAN LIFE?

I
THE BENEFIT TO HUMANITY

Complaints of the shortness of our life.—Theory of " medical selection " as a cause of degeneration of the race.—Utility of prolonging human life 132

II

SUGGESTIONS FOR THE PROLONGATION OF LIFE

Ancient methods of prolonging human life.—Gerokomy.—The "immortality draught" of the Taoists.—Brown-Séquard's method.—The spermine of Poehl.—Dr. Weber's precepts.—Increased duration of life in historical times.—Hygienic maxims.—Decrease in cutaneous cancer 136

III

DISEASES THAT SHORTEN LIFE

Measures against infectious diseases as aiding in the prolongation of life.—Prevention of syphilis.—Attempts to prepare serums which could strengthen the higher elements of the organism 145

IV

INTESTINAL PUTREFACTION SHORTENS LIFE

Uselessness of the large intestine in man.—Case of a woman whose large intestine was inactive for six months.—Another case where the greater part of the large intestine was completely shut off.—Attempts to disinfect the contents of the large intestine.—Prolonged mastication as a means of preventing intestinal putrefaction 151

V

LACTIC ACID AS INHIBITING INTESTINAL PUTREFACTION

The development of the intestinal flora in man.—Harmlessness of sterilised food.—Means of preventing the putrefaction of food.—Lactic fermentation and its anti-putrescent action.—Experiments on man and mice.—Longevity in races which used soured milk.—Comparative study of different soured milks.—Properties of the Bulgarian Bacillus.—Means of preventing intestinal putrefaction with the help of microbes 161

PART V
PSYCHICAL RUDIMENTS IN MAN

I

RUDIMENTARY ORGANS IN MAN

Reply to critics who deny the simian origin of man.—Actual existence of rudimentary organs.—Reductions in the struc-

# CONTENTS

ture of the organs of sense in man.—Atrophy of Jacobson's organ and of the Harderian gland in the human race . . 184

II

HUMAN TRAITS OF CHARACTER INHERITED FROM APES

The mental character of anthropoid apes.—Their muscular strength.—Their expression of fear.—The awakening of latent instincts of man under the influence of fear . . 191

III

SOMNAMBULISM AND HYSTERIA AS MENTAL RELICS

Fear as the primary cause of hysteria.—Natural somnambulism.—Doubling of personality.—Some examples of somnambulists.—Analogy between somnambulism and the life of anthropoid apes.—The psychology of crowds.—Importance of the investigation of hysteria for the problem of the origin of man 200

PART VI
SOME POINTS IN THE HISTORY OF SOCIAL ANIMALS

I

THE INDIVIDUAL AND THE RACE

Problem of the species in the human race.—Loss of individuality in the associations of lower animals.—Myxomycetes and Siphonophora.—Individuality in Ascidians.—Progress in the development of the individual living in a society . . 212

II

INSECT SOCIETIES

Social life of insects.—Development and preservation of individuality in colonies of insects.—Division of labour and sacrifice of individuality in some insects 220

III

SOCIETY AND THE INDIVIDUAL IN THE HUMAN RACE

Human societies.—Differentiation in the human race.—Learned women.—Habits of a bee, *Halictus quadricinctus*.—Collectivist theories.—Criticisms by Herbert Spencer and

CONTENTS

Nietzsche.—Progress of individuality in the societies of higher beings 223

PART VII
PESSIMISM AND OPTIMISM

I
PREVALENCE OF PESSIMISM

Oriental origin of pessimism.—Pessimistic poets.—Byron.—Leopardi.—Poushkin.—Lermontoff.—Pessimism and suicide 233

II
ANALYSIS OF PESSIMISM

Attempts to assign reasons for the pessimistic conception of life.—Views of E. von Hartmann.—Analysis of Kowalevsky's work on the psychology of pessimism 239

III
PESSIMISM IN ITS RELATION TO HEALTH AND AGE

Relation between pessimism and the state of the health.—History of a man of science who was pessimistic when young and who became an optimist in old age.—Optimism of Schopenhauer when old.—Development of the sense of life.—Development of the senses in blind people.—The sense of obstacles 247

PART VIII
GOETHE AND FAUST

I
GOETHE'S YOUTH

Goethe's youth.—Pessimism of youth.—Werther.—Tendency to suicide.—Work and love.—Goethe's conception of life in his maturity 261

II
GOETHE AND OPTIMISM

Goethe's optimistic period.—His mode of life in that period.—Influence of love in artistic production.—Inclinations towards the arts must be regarded as secondary sexual char-

CONTENTS

acters.—Senile love of Goethe.—Relation between genius and the sexual activities 270

III
GOETHE'S OLD AGE

Old age of Goethe.—Physical and intellectual vigour of the old man.—Optimistic conception of life.—Happiness in life in his last period 279

IV
GOETHE AND " FAUST "

Faust the biography of Goethe.—The three monologues in the first Part.—Faust's pessimism.—The brain-fatigue which finds a remedy in love.—The romance with Marguerite and its unhappy ending 283

V
THE OLD AGE OF FAUST

The second Part of *Faust* is in the main a description of senile love.—Amorous passion of the old man.—Humble attitude of the old Faust.—Platonic love for Helena.—The old Faust's conception of life.—His optimism.—The general idea of the play 290

PART IX
SCIENCE AND MORALITY
I
UTILITARIAN AND INTUITIVE MORALITY

Difficulty of the problem of morality.—Vivisection and anti-vivisection.—Enquiry into the possibility of rational morality.—Utilitarian and intuitive theories of morality.—Insufficiency of these 301

II
MORALITY AND HUMAN NATURE

Attempts to found morality on the laws of human nature.—Kant's theory of moral obligation.—Some criticisms of the Kantian theory.—Moral conduct must be guided by reason 309

III

INDIVIDUALISM

Individual morality.—History of two brothers brought up in the same circumstances, but whose conduct was quite different.—Late development of the sense of life.—Evolution of sympathy.—The sphere of egoism in moral conduct.—Christian morality.—Morality of Herbert Spencer.—Danger of exalted altruism 316

IV

ORTHOBIOSIS

Human nature must be modified according to an ideal.—Comparison with the modification of the constitution of plants and of animals.—Schlanstedt rye.—Burbank's plants.—The ideal of orthobiosis.—The immorality of ignorance.—The place of hygiene in the social life.—The place of altruism in moral conduct.—The freedom of the theory of orthobiosis from metaphysics 325

THE PROLONGATION OF LIFE

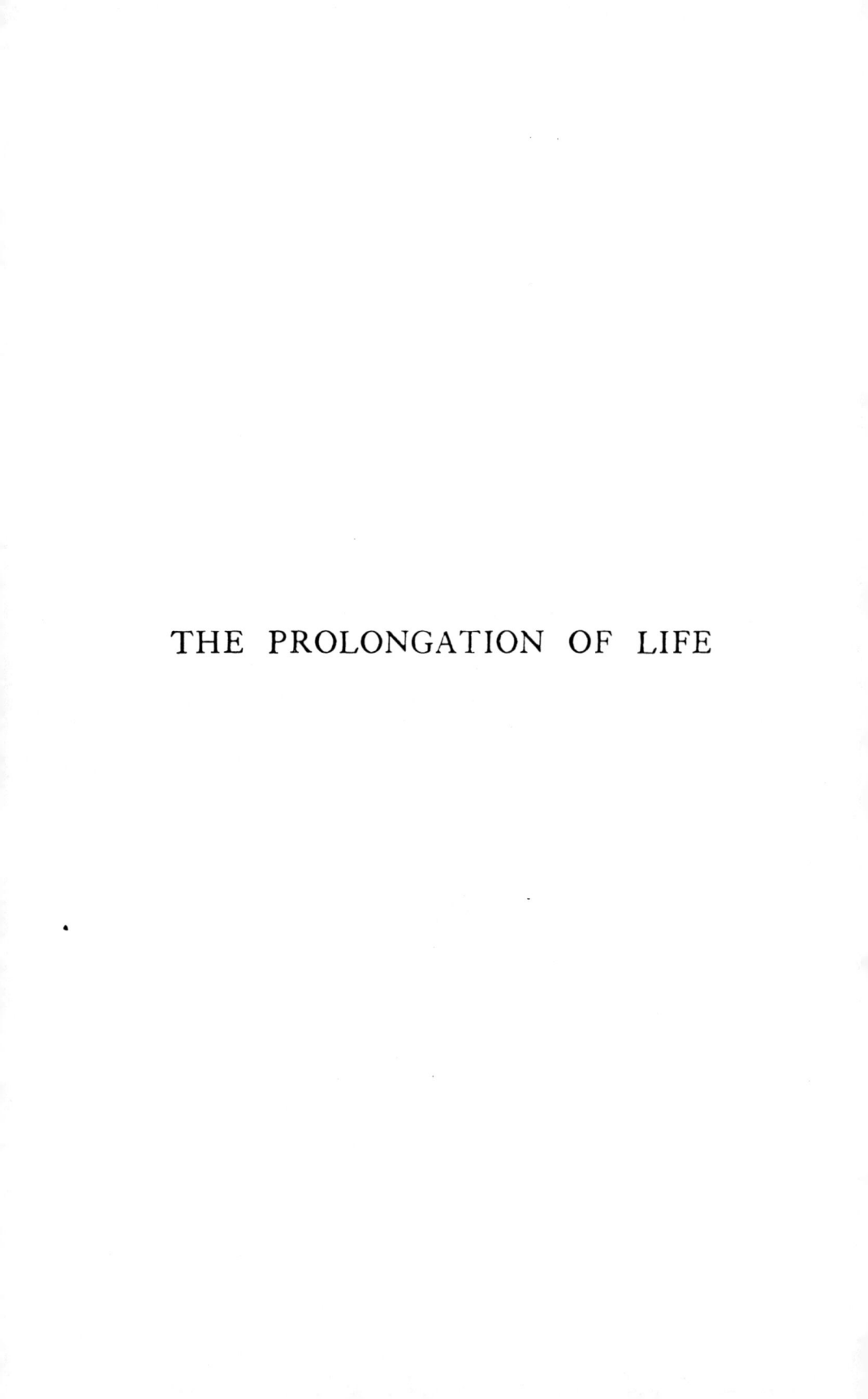

PART I

THE INVESTIGATION OF OLD AGE

1

THE PROBLEMS OF SENILITY

Treatment of old people in uncivilised countries—Assassination of old people in civilised countries—Suicide of old people—Public assistance in old age—Centenarians—Mme. Robineau, a lady of 106 years of age—Principal characters of old age—Examples of old mammals—Old birds and tortoises—Hypothesis of senile degeneration in the lower animals

In the " Nature of Man " I laid down the outlines of a theory of the actual changes which take place during the senescence of our body. These ideas, on the one hand, have raised certain difficulties, and, on the other, have led to new investigations. As the study of old age is of great theoretical importance, and naturally is of practical value, I think that it is useful to pursue the subject still further.

Although there exist races which solve the difficulty of old age by the simple means of destroying aged people, the problem in civilised countries is complicated by our more refined feelings and by considerations of a general nature.

In the Melanesian Islands, old people who have become incapable of doing useful work are buried alive.

In times of famine, the natives of Tierra del Fuego kill and eat the old women before they touch their dogs.

When they were asked why they did this, they said that dogs could catch seals, whilst old women could not do so.

Civilised races do not act like the Fuegians or other savages; they neither kill nor eat the aged, but none the less life in old age often becomes very sad. As they are incapable of performing any useful function in the family or in the village, the old people are regarded as a heavy burden. Although they cannot be got rid of, their death is awaited with eagerness, and is never thought to come soon enough. The Italians say that old women have seven lives. According to a Bergamask tradition, old women have seven souls, and after that an eighth soul, quite a little one, and after that again half a soul; whilst the Lithuanians complain that the life of an old woman is so tough that it cannot be crushed even in a mill. We may take it as an echo of such popular ideas that murders of old people are extremely common even in the most civilised European countries. I have been astonished in looking through criminal records to see how many cases there are of the murder of old people, specially of old women. It is easy to divine the motives of these acts. A convict of the Island of Saghalien, condemned for the assassination of several old persons, declared naïvely to the prison doctor: "Why pity them? They were already old, and would have died in any case in a few years."

In the celebrated novel of Dostoiewsky, "Crime and Punishment," there is a tavern scene where young people discuss all sorts of general topics. In the middle of the conversation a student declares that he would " murder and rob any cursed old woman without the least remorse." " If the truth were told," he goes on to say, "this is how I look at the thing. On the one hand a stupid old woman, childish, worthless, ill-tempered, and in bad health; no one would miss her, indeed she is a nuisance to everyone. She does not even herself know any reason why she should live, and perhaps to-morrow death will make a good riddance of her. On the other hand, there are fresh and vigorous young people who are dying in their thousands, in the most senseless way, no one troubling about them, and everywhere the same thing is going on."

Old people not only run the risk of murder; they very often end their own lives prematurely by suicide.

They prefer death to a life oppressed by material hardships or burdened by diseases. The daily papers give many instances of old people who, tired of suffering, asphyxiate themselves by their charcoal stoves.

The frequency of suicide in the case of the old has been established by numerous statistics, and the new facts which I now cite do no more than confirm it. In 1878, in Prussia, amongst 100,000 individuals there were 154 cases of suicide of men between the ages of 20 and 50, but 295, that is to say, nearly twice as many of men between the ages of 50 and 80. In Denmark, a country in which suicide is notoriously common, a similar proportion exists. Thus, in Copenhagen, in the ten years from 1886 to 1895, there were 394 suicides of men between 50 and 70. These figures relate to 100,000 individuals. Of the suicides $36\frac{1}{2}$ per cent. were those of people in the prime of life, $63\frac{1}{2}$ per cent. those of the aged.[1]

In such circumstances, it is natural that politicians and philanthropists have made many attempts to ameliorate the old age of the poor. In some countries laws have been passed to bring about this. For instance, a Danish law of June 27th, 1891, established compulsory aid for the aged, enacting that every person more than 60 years old was to have the legal right to aid if required. In 1896 more than 36,000 people (36,246) were pensioned

[1] Westergaard, *Mortalitaet u. Morbilitaet*, 2nd. Edit., 1901, pp. 653-655.

under this law, at a cost of nearly £200,000. In Belgium, the indigent old people are not pensioned until they reach the age of 65. In France, until recently, the aged poor could be supported at the public expense only by prosecuting them and sending them to prison for begging. This state of affairs, however, ceased with the application of the law of July 15th, 1905, according to which any French subject without resources, unable to support himself by work, and either more than 70 years of age, or suffering from some incurable infirmity or disease, is to receive public assistance.

It has been thought the proper course to make such laws, and to lay the burden on the general population, without inquiring if it may not be possible to retard the debility of old age to such an extent that very old people might still be able to earn their livelihood by work. Old age can be studied by the methods of exact science, and there may yet be established some regimen by which health and vigour will be preserved beyond the age where now it is generally necessary to resort to public charity. With this object, a systematic investigation of senescence should be made in institutions for the aged, where there are always a large number of people from 75 to 90 years old, although centenarians are extremely rare. I know many institutions for aged men where, from their first foundation, there has been no case of an inhabitant reaching the age of 100, and even in similar institutions for women, although women live to much greater ages than men, centenarians are very rare. At the Salpêtrière, for instance, where there is always a large number of old women, it is the rarest chance to find a centenarian. Opportunity for the study of the extremely aged is to be found only in private families.

THE PROBLEMS OF SENILITY

Most of the centenarians whom I have been able to see have been so defective mentally that all that can be studied in them are the physical qualities and functions. A few years ago an old woman who had reached her 100th year was the pride of the Salpêtrière. She was bedridden and extremely feeble physically and mentally. She replied briefly when she was asked questions, but apparently without any idea of what they meant.

Not long ago, a lady who lived in a suburb of Rouen reached her 100th birthday. The local newspapers wrote exaggerated articles about her, praising the integrity of her mind and her physical strength. I paid a visit to her myself, hoping to make a detailed investigation, but I found at once that the journalists had completely misrepresented her condition. Although her physical health was fairly good, her intelligence had degenerated to such an extent that I had to abandon the idea of any serious investigation.

The most interesting of all the centenarians with whom I have become acquainted had reached an extremely advanced age, having entered upon her 107th year. It is about two years ago that a journalist, Monsieur Flamans, took me to see this Mme. Robineau who lived in a suburb of Paris. I found her a very old-looking lady, rather short, thin, with a bent back, and leaning heavily on a cane when she walked. The physical condition (Mme. Robineau was born on January 12th, 1800), of this woman of more than 106 years, showed extreme decay. She had only one tooth; she had to sit down after every few steps, but, once comfortably seated, she could remain in that position for quite a long time. She went to bed early and got up very late. Her features displayed very great age (see Fig. 1), although her skin was not extremely wrinkled.

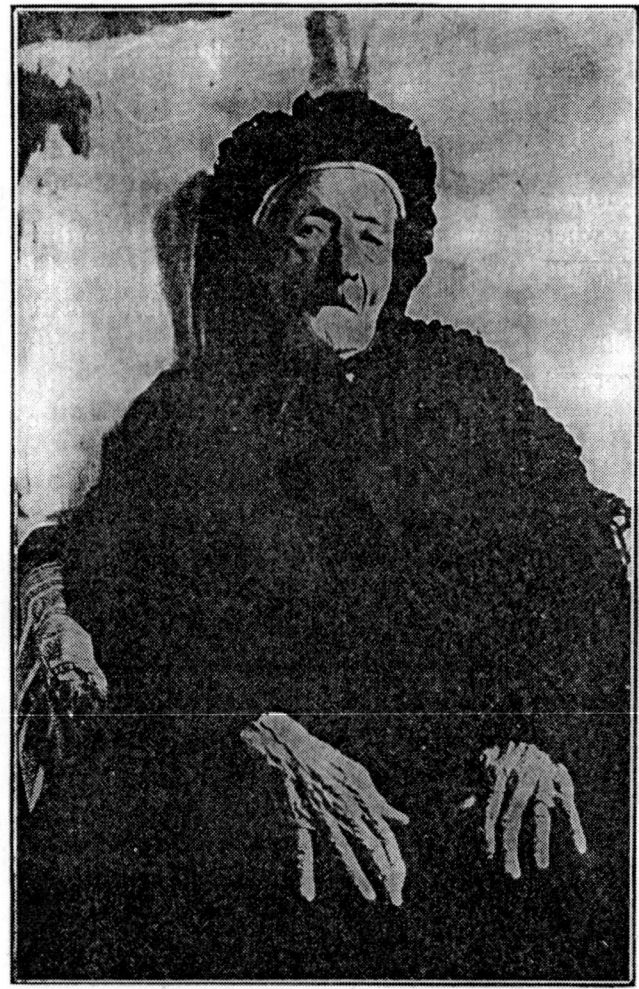

FIG. 1.—Mme. Robineau, a centenarian. From a photograph taken on her one hundred and fifth birthday.

The skin of her hands had become so transparent that one could see the bones, the blood-vessels, and the tendons. Her senses were very feeble; she could see only with one eye; taste and smell were extremely rudimentary; her hearing was her best means of relation with the external world. None the less, Dr. Löwenberg, a well-known aurist, had assured himself that her auditory organs showed in a most marked degree, the usual signs of old age, such as complete insensibility to high notes and slight deafness for low notes. Dr. Löwenberg attributed these changes to senile degeneration of the ear which affected more and more seriously the nervous mechanism although it had caused little change in the conducting apparatus. Notwithstanding her physical weakness, Mme. Robineau retained her intelligence fully, her mind remained delicate and refined and the goodness of her heart was touching. In contrast with the usual selfishness of old people, Mme. Robineau took a vivid interest in those around her. Her conversation was intelligent, connected, and logical. Examination of the physical functions of this old lady revealed facts of great interest. Dr. Ambard found that the sounds of the heart were normal, but perhaps a little accentuated. The pulse was regular, 70 to 84 a minute, and its tension was normal. The arterial pressure was 17. The lungs were sound. All these facts testify to her general health. The most remarkable circumstance was the absence of sclerosis of the arteries, although such degeneration is usually believed to be a normal character of old age.

Analysis of the urine, made on several occasions, showed that the kidneys were affected with a chronic disease, which, however, was not serious.[1]

Although the sense of taste was weak, Madame Robineau

[1] The volume of the urine excreted in 24 hours (in January 1905) was 500 c.c., with a density of 1019. There was no albumen or sugar. The quantity, per litre, of urea was 11·50 gr., of chlorides 9 gr., of phosphates 1·15 gr. The sediment contained crystals of uric acid, some pavement epithelium cells, a very few cells from the tubules, some hyaline platelets and isolated white corpuscles.

had a fair appetite. She ate and drank little, but her diet was varied. She took butcher's meat or chicken extremely seldom, but ate eggs, fish, farinaceous food, vegetables, and stewed fruit, and drank sweetened water with a little white wine, and sometimes, after a meal, a small glass of dessert wine. The processes of alimentary digestion and excretion were normal.

It has sometimes been thought that duration of life is a hereditary property. There was no evidence for this in the present case. Madame Robineau's relatives had died comparatively early in life, and a centenarian was unknown in her family. Her great age was an acquired character. Her whole life had been extremely regular. She had married a timber merchant, and had lived for many years in a suburb of Paris in comfortable circumstances. Her character was gentle and affectionate; she was thoroughly domesticated, and had been devoted to home life with very few distractions.

At the age of 106 years, her intelligence suddenly became weak. She lost her memory almost completely, and sometimes wandered. But her gentle and affectionate disposition remained unaltered.

The appearance of aged persons is too well known to make detailed description necessary. The skin of the face is dry and wrinkled and generally pale; the hairs on the head and the body are white; the back is bent, and the gait is slow and laborious, whilst the memory is weak. Such are the most familiar traits of old age. Baldness is not a special character; it often begins during youth and naturally is progressive, but if it has not already appeared, it does not come on with old age.

The stature diminishes in old age. As the result of a series of observations, it has been established that a man loses more than an inch (3·166 cm.), and a woman than an inch and a half (4·3 cm.), between the ages of fifty and eighty-five years. In extreme cases, the loss may be nearly three inches. The weight also becomes less. According to Quételet, males attain their maximum weights at the age of forty, females at that of fifty. From the age of sixty years onwards, the body becomes lighter, the loss at eighty being as much as thirteen pounds.

Such losses of height and weight are signs of the general atrophy of the aged organism. Not merely the soft parts, such as the muscles and viscera, but even the bones lose weight, in the latter case the loss being of the mineral constituents. This process of decalcification makes the skeleton brittle, and is sometimes the cause of fatal accidents.

The loss of muscular tissue is specially great. The volume diminishes, and the substance becomes paler; the fat between the fibres is absorbed, and may disappear completely. Movements are slower, and the muscular force is abated. This progressive degeneration has been examined by dynamometrical measurements of the hand and the trunk, and is greater in males than in females.

The volumes and weights of the visceral organs similarly become smaller, but the diminution is not uniform.

The old age of lower mammals presents characters similar to those found in man. I can now give other instances than the case of the old dog which I described in the " Nature of Man."

I will first take the case of old elephants, described by a competent observer. "The general appearance is wretched, the skull being often hardly covered with skin; there are deep abrasions under the eyes, and smaller ones on the cheeks, whilst the skin of the forehead is very often deeply fissured or covered with lumps. The eyes are usually dim, and discharge an abnormal quantity of water. The margin of the ears, specially on the lower side, is usually frayed. The skin of the trunk is roughened, hard, and warty, so that the organ has lost much of its flexibility. The skin on the body generally is worn and wrinkled; the legs are thinner than in maturity, the

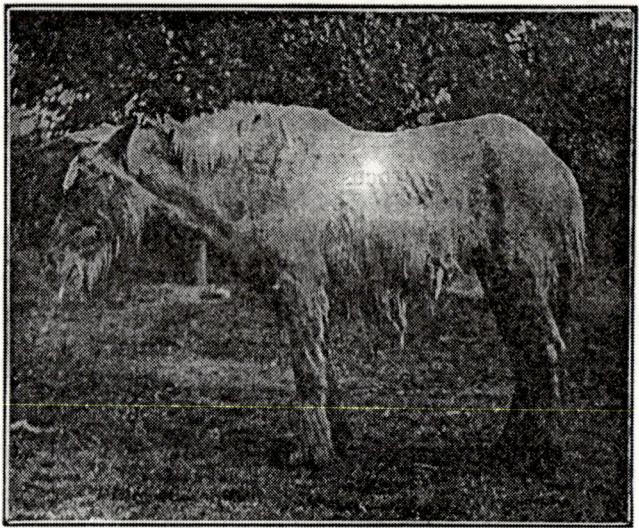

FIG. 2.—A Mare, thirty-seven years old.

huge mass of muscles being much shrunken, whilst the circumference, especially just above the feet, is considerably reduced. The skin round the toe-nails is roughened and frayed. The tail is scaly and hard, and the tip is often hairless.

Horses begin to grow old much sooner than elephants. I reproduce (Fig. 2) the photograph of a rare instance of longevity, a mare 37 years old, which belonged to M.

THE PROBLEMS OF SENILITY

Métaine, in the department of Mayenne. The skin, bare in places, but elsewhere covered with long hairs, shows considerable atrophy. The general attitude reveals the feebleness of the whole body. Many birds, on the other hand, show at similar ages very slight external change, as may be seen from the photograph of a duck more than 25 years old (Fig. 3) which belonged to Dr. Jean Charcot. At a still greater age, as may be seen occasionally in parrots,

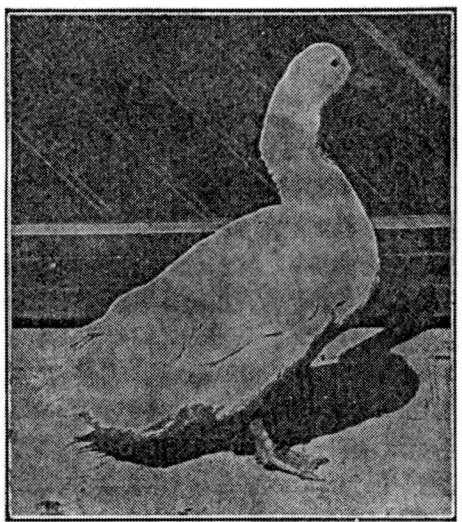

FIG. 3.—A White Duck, which lived for more than a quarter of a century.

the general debility of the body reveals itself in the attitude, in the condition of the feathers, and in the swelling of the joints. On the other hand, the oldest reptiles which have been observed do not differ in appearance from normal adults of the same species. I have in my possession a male tortoise (*Testudo mauritanica*) given me by my friends MM. Rabaud and Caullery, and which is at least 86 years old. It shows no sign of old age, and in all respects behaves like any other individual of this species. More than 31 years ago it was wounded by a blow, the traces of which remain visible on the right side of the carapace (Fig. 4). In the last three years the tortoise lived in a garden at Montauban, along with two females which laid fertile eggs. The old male, although, as I have said, probably at least 86 years of age, was still sexually healthy.

I have borrowed from the interesting volume of Prof. Sir E. Ray Lankester[1] the figure (Fig. 5) and de-

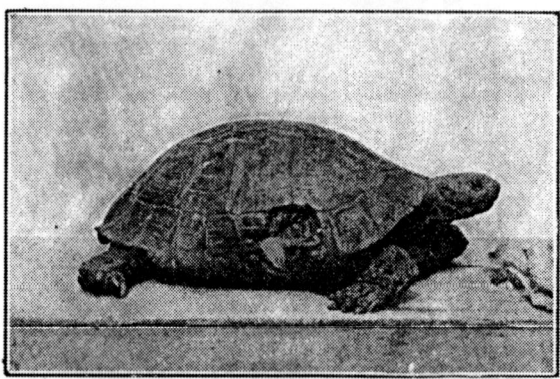

FIG. 4.—An Old Land-tortoise.

scription of a giant tortoise from the island of Mauritius, which is probably the oldest of all living animals. It was brought to Mauritius from the Seychelles in 1764, and has lived since then in the garden of the Governor, and as it has thus already been 140 years in captivity, its age must be at least 150 years, although we have not exact information. Notwithstanding this, it shows no signs of old age.

The examples which I have brought together show that

[1] *Extinct Animals*, London, 1905, pp. 28, 29.

often amongst vertebrates there are some animals the organisms of which withstand the ravages of time much better than that of man. I think it a fair inference that senility, the precocious senescence which is one of the greatest sorrows of humanity, is not so profoundly seated in the constitution of the higher animals as has generally been supposed. It is not necessary, therefore, to discuss at

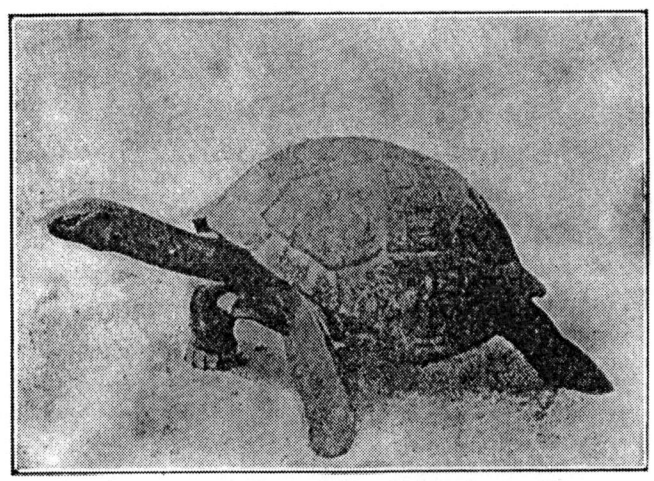

FIG. 5.—A Water-tortoise, more than 150 years old.
(After Prof. Sir E. Ray Lankester.)

length the general question as to whether senile degeneration is an inevitable event in living organisms.

I have already shown, in the "Nature of Man," the difference which exists between senile degeneration in our own bodies and the phenomena of senescence amongst Infusoria which, as M. Maupas described, are followed by a process of rejuvenescence. According to the more recent results of several investigators, the difference is still greater than I had supposed. Enriquez[1] has been able

[1] *Rendiconti d. Accad. d. Lincei*, 1906, vol xiv. pp. 351, 390.

to propagate Infusoria to the 700th generation without any sign of senility being displayed. Here we are far from the condition in the human race.

R. Hertwig,[1] one of the best observers of the lower animals, has recently attempted to show that the very simple animalculæ of the genus *Actinosphaerium* are subject to true physiological degeneration. He has several times seen cultures of this Rhizopod degenerate, until all the individuals had died, notwithstanding the presence of abundant food. Prof. Hertwig attributed this to the "constitution of the *Actinosphaerium* having been weakened by too great vital activity at an earlier stage." I should have thought that it was a much more natural explanation to suppose that the culture had undergone infection by one of the contagious diseases which so often destroy cultures of different kinds of lower animals and plants. As this idea had not occurred to the observer, he had not searched for parasitic microbes amongst the granulations which are always present in the body of an *Actinosphaerium*. However this may be, I cannot accept the facts brought forward by this distinguished German as a valid proof of the existence of senile degeneration in these lowly creatures.

The facts that I have brought together in this chapter justify the conclusion that human beings who reach extreme old age may preserve their mental qualities notwithstanding serious physical decay. Moreover, it is equally plain that the organism of some vertebrates is able to resist the influence of time much longer than is the case with man under present conditions.

[1] *Ueb. d. physiologische Degeneration bei Actinosphaerium eichhornii.* Jena, 1904.

II

THEORIES OF CAUSATION OF SENILITY

Hypothesis of the causation of senility—Senility cannot be attributed to the cessation of the power of reproduction of the cells of the body—Growth of the hair and the nails in old age—Inner mechanism of the senescence of the tissues—Notwithstanding the criticisms of M. Marinesco, the neuronophags are true phagocytes—The whitening of hair and the destruction of nerve cells, as arguments against a theory of old age based on the failure of the reproductive powers of the cells

ALTHOUGH it has not been proved that living matter must inevitably undergo senile decrepitude, it is none the less true that man and his nearest allies generally exhibit such degeneration. It is therefore extremely important to recognise the real causes of our senescence. There have been many hypotheses on the subject, but there are comparatively few definite facts known.

Bütschli has supposed that the life of cells is maintained by a specific vital ferment which becomes feebler in proportion to the extent of cellular reproduction, but I cannot regard this as more than a pious opinion. The ferment has never been seen, and we do not know of its actual existence. According to the better-known theory of Prof. Weismann, old age depends on a limitation in the power of cells to reproduce, so that a time comes when the body can no longer replace the wastage of cells which is an inevitable accompaniment of life As old age appears at different times in different species and different individuals, Weismann has concluded that the possible number of cell generations differs in different cases. He has not found, however, a solution of the problem as to why multiplication of cells should cease in one individual, whereas it proceeds much further in other individuals. Prof. Minot,[1] the American zoologist, has developed a similar theory, and has employed an exact method to determine the gradual diminution in the rate of growth of an animal from its birth onwards. According to him, the power of reproduction of the cells weakens progressively during life, until a point is necessarily reached at which the organism, no longer capable of repairing itself, begins to atrophy and degenerate. Dr. Buehler[2] has recently laid stress upon this theory.

There is no doubt that cells reproduce much more actively during the embryonic period. The process becomes slower later on, but, none the less, continues to display itself throughout the whole period of life. Buehler attributes the difficulty with which certain wounds heal in the case of old people to the insufficiency of cellular reproduction. He thinks in particular that the proliferation of the cells of the skin, to replace those which are worn off from the surface, becomes less active with age. According to him, it is theoretically obvious that a time must come when the replacement of the epidermic cells completely ceases. As the superficial layers of the skin continue to dry up and be cast off, it is plain that the epidermis must disappear completely. Buehler thinks that there must be

[1] "Senescence and Rejuvenation," *Journal of Physiology*, 1891, t. xii.
[2] *Biologisches Centralblatt*, 1904, pp. 65, 81, 113.

THEORIES OF CAUSATION OF SENILITY

a similar fate for the genital glands, the muscles, and all the other organs.

These theoretical considerations, however, are not compatible with certain well-known facts indicating that there is no general cessation of the power of cell reproduction in old age. The hairs and the nails, which are epidermic outgrowths, continue to grow throughout life, their growth being due to the proliferation of their constituent cells. There is no sign of any arrest in the development of these structures, even in the most advanced old age. The reverse is true. It is well known that the hairs on some parts of the body increase in number and in length in old people. In some lower races, for instance in the Mongols, the moustache and the beard grow vigorously in old age, whilst young people of the same race have only very small moustaches and practically no trace of beard. So also in white women the fine and almost invisible down which covers the upper lip, the chin, and the cheeks in the young may become replaced by long hairs which form a moustache or beard.

Dr. Pohl, a specialist in the growth of hair, has measured the rate of growth in different circumstances. He has shown that in an old man of 61 the hair on the temple grew 11 mm. in a month; on the other hand, the hair on the same region in boys of 11 to 15 years old grew in the same time only from 11 to 12 mm. Plainly, there is no case here of a progressive diminution of cell-proliferation with age. The same observer, it is true, has shown that the hair of young men of between 21 and 24 years grew at the rate of 15 mm. a month, whilst in the same individuals, at the age of 61 years, the rate of growth was only 11 mm.; but this diminution in the rate of growth is only apparent. The first figure concerned the hair taken from different regions of the scalp, whilst the second related only to the hair on the temples, and Dr. Pohl himself has shown that, in the latter region, the hair grows slower than in other regions. Moreover, in many boys of 11 to 15 years old, studied by this observer, the rate of growth was always less than 15 mm., and often less even than the 11 mm. recorded in the old man of 61.

I have been able to note that the nails grow even in very old people. In the case of Mme. Robineau, the centenarian, the nail of the middle finger of the left hand grew $2\frac{1}{2}$ mm. in three weeks. In the case of a lady of 32 years old, the corresponding nail grew 3 mm. in two weeks, the difference being out of all proportion to the enormous difference in the age. The centenarian's nails had to be cut from time to time.

Although the hairs of old people grow, they become white, which is a phenomenon of senile degeneration. Although they increase in length, the colouring matter in them becomes reduced and finally disappears. In the "Nature of Man" I described the process by which this blanching takes place, and which may now be regarded as definitely proved. It is useful as a means of interpreting the real nature of the process of senescence. In several published works, I have explained my belief that just as the pigment of the hair is destroyed by phagocytes, so also the atrophy of other organs of the body, in old age, is very frequently due to the action of devouring cells which I have called macrophags. These are the phagocytes that destroy the higher elements of the body, such as the nervous and muscular cells, and the cells of the liver and kidneys. This part of my theory has encountered very strong criticism, especially with regard to the part played by the macrophags in the senescence of nervous tissue.

THEORIES OF CAUSATION OF SENILITY

Neurologists in particular, have criticised my interpretation. For several years M. Marinesco[1] has attacked my theory of the atrophy of the nerve-cells in old age. In the first place, he has stated that in old people, and even if these are very old, it is rare to find phagocytes surrounding and devouring the cells of the brain. In support of this contention, he has been good enough to send me two preparations made from the brains of two very old persons. After careful examination I was convinced that my opponent had been inexact. In the brain of the two centenarians (one of whom died at the age of 117 years) there were very many nerve-cells surrounded by phagocytes and in process of being destroyed by them. It happened, however, that as the sections were very weakly stained, it was more difficult to observe the facts than in the preparations upon which I had made my own observations. I have already recorded this fact in the second and third French editions of the "Nature of Man."

Without taking notice of my reply, M. Marinesco has published another criticism of my theory in an article[2] entitled "Histological Investigations into the Mechanism of Senility." In that work, although he himself had invented the designation "neuronophag" for a phagocyte that devours nerve-cells, he denies the existence of such a power. He thinks that nerve-cells atrophy independently of the cells that surround them. The latter, the so-called neuronophags, only contribute to the atrophy inasmuch as they press against the nerve-cells and deprive them of nutrition. He is confident that the constituent parts of nerve-cells are never found in the neuronophags. There is no question of

---

[1] *Comptes rendus de l'Académie des sciences*, 23 April, 1900.
[2] *Revue générale des sciences*, 30 Dec., 1904, p. 1116.

phagocytosis, of the existence of cells that devour their neighbours.

M. Léri has taken a similar view in a Report on the Senile Brain[1] presented to a recent congress of alienists and neurologists. According to him "the nuclei which surround some of the atrophying nerve-cells do not play the part of neuronophags." In his monograph "La Neuronophagie,"[2] M. Sand elaborates the same view. He relies on his observation that "neuronophags are usually either devoid of protoplasm or display only a very thin layer of it. They never exhibit protoplasmic outgrowths, and they never have granules in their cellular bodies (p. 86)." Still more recently MM. Laignel-Lavastine and Voisin[3] have taken the same view, maintaining that the neuronophags do not display phagocytosis.

Although I cannot undertake here to give a detailed reply to the arguments of my critics, I may point out a fallacy that vitiates their reasoning. The study of the intimate structure of nervous tissue involves the treatment of that very delicate substance by numerous active reagents. It is extremely important not to forget the possibility of alterations which may be produced in the processes of preparation and which are extremely difficult to avoid. A glance at the figures given by my critics shows me that the neuronophags in their preparations had been subjected to violent treatment. When M. Léri speaks of "the nuclei which surround some of the nerve-cells," and M. Sand of "cells without protoplasm," it is clear that they had been observing cells destroyed by the processes of the laboratory. The

[1] *Le Bulletin médical*, 1906, p. 721; *Le Cerveau sénile*, Lille, 1906, pp. 64-69.

[2] *Mémoires couronnés publiés par l'Académie royale de Belgique*, Bruxelles, 1906.

[3] *Revue de Médecine*, Nov., 1906, p. 870.

THEORIES OF CAUSATION OF SENILITY

illustrations in the memoir of M. Marinesco show that in his preparations, too, the neuronophags had been very greatly altered.

It is well known that nuclei do not exist free in tissues, and that when they appear devoid of protoplasm, there has been some defect in the technical methods of preparing them for examination. As a matter of fact, neuronophags do not consist of nuclei with at the most a pellicle of protoplasm; like other cells, they have protoplasmic bodies which, however, are frequently destroyed by the violent processes of histological preparation.

The arguments of my critics recall to me the words of a medical student, who, on being asked to describe the microbe of tuberculosis, said that it was a little red bacillus. The bacillus in question, like most bacilli, is colourless, but it is usual to stain it so that it may be visible under the microscope. The student, knowing it only in particular preparations, had a false idea of its appearance.

In well-made preparations, neuronophags are typical cells with abundant protoplasm. When they have been preserved by a process that does not dissolve their contents, they show granules like those found in nerve-cells.

To study neuronophagy, M. Manouélian,[1] in the laboratory of the Pasteur Institute in Paris, set himself to improve the technical methods of preparation. He succeeded in showing first that in the destruction of nerve-cells that occurs in cases of hydrophobia, the contents of these cells are absorbed by the surrounding neuronophags. "My observations on the cerebro-spinal ganglia of human cases of hydrophobia," he wrote; "show clearly that the macrophags act as phagocytes of the nerve-cells." "Most of the cells in the nerve-ganglia contain yellow, brown, and black

[1] *Annales de l'Institut Pasteur*, Oct. 1906, p. 859.

pigmented granules, usually united in small masses. What becomes of these granulations on the destruction and disappearance of the nerve-cell? If, as M. Marinesco has it, there is no phagocytosis by the surrounding cells, but merely a mechanical interference, then the granules, on the destruction of the nerve-cells that contained them, should be found lying in the interstitial tissue. But this does not happen. The granules are ingested by cells which are true macrophags."

By the aid of a very delicate mode of preparation, M. Manouélian has shown that in the case of senile brains the granules of the nerve-cells are absorbed by neuronophags. I have myself studied M. Manouélian's preparations and can testify to the accuracy of his observations (Figs. 6 and 7).

Doubt is no longer possible. In senile degeneration the nerve-cells are surrounded by neuronophags which absorb their contents and bring about more or less complete atrophy. It has been supposed that in order to devour their contents, the neuronophags must penetrate the nerve-cells, and such an event has rarely been seen. But it is well known, the phagocytosis of red blood corpuscles being a typical instance, that to absorb a cell a phagocyte does not necessarily engulf it bodily or penetrate it, but may gradually denude it of its contents merely by resting in contact with it.

There has been some discussion as to the condition of nerve-cells which are on the point of being devoured by neuronophags. It has been noticed that such cells may display a considerable amount of degeneration without being devoured, whilst, on the other hand, cells apparently normal have been found undergoing phagocytosis. As I cannot state definitely what are the conditions that induce

THEORIES OF CAUSATION OF SENILITY

the phagocytosis of nerve-cells, I shall not attempt a discussion of the problem.

Although the destruction of nerve-cells by neuronophags is a general occurrence in senile brains, one may conceive of cases where this does not occur. And so, in old people who have preserved their faculties, it may well be that the neuronophags have refrained from attacking the nerve-cells.

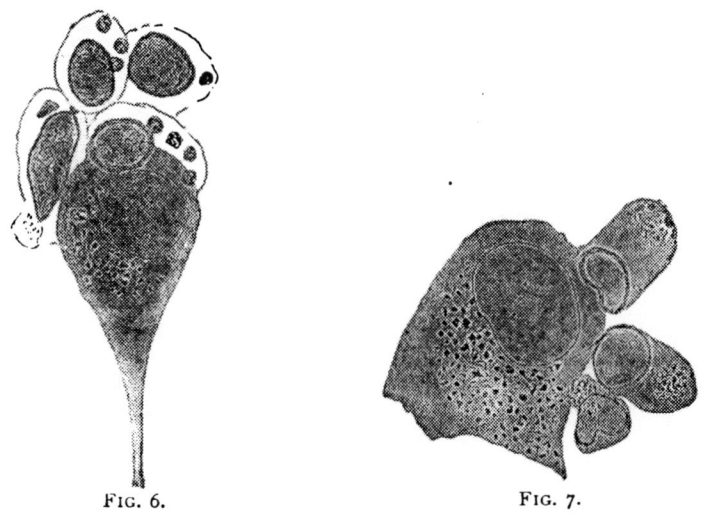

FIG. 6.   FIG. 7.

FIGS. 6. & 7.—Two nerve-cells from the cortex of the brain of an old dog aged fifteen years.
The neuronophags surrounding the nerve-cells contain numerous granulations.
(From preparations made by M. Manouélian.)

But as such instances are rare, so also phagocytosis is usually found in senile brains, and I cannot accept M. Sand's denial of its existence, based on his study of two cases.

The general result of my investigation into the criticisms that have been published on this matter has confirmed me in my belief that neuronophagy plays a most important part in senescence, and recent observations that I have made with M. Weinberg have completely supported this view.

The bleaching of hair and the atrophy of the brain in old age thus furnish important arguments against the view that senescence is the result of arrest of the reproductive powers of cells. Hairs grow old and become white without ceasing to grow. The cessation of the power of reproduction cannot be the cause of the senescence of brain-cells, for these cells do not reproduce even in youth.

III

MECHANISM OF SENILITY

Action of the macrophags in destroying the higher cells—Senile degeneration of muscular fibres—Atrophy of the skeleton—Atheroma and arterial sclerosis—Theory that old age is due to alteration in the vascular glands—Organic tissues that resist phagocytosis

THE instances which I have selected in attempting to describe the mechanism of senescence of the tissues are not the only cases in which the importance of phagocytosis is evident. The blanching of hair is due to the destructive agency of chromophags; in atrophy of the brain neuronophags destroy the higher nerve-cells. In addition to these instances of phagocytosis, in which the active agents belong to the category of macrophags, there are many other devouring cells, adrift in the tissues of the aged, and ready to cause destruction of other cells of the higher type. The phagocytic action is not so manifest as in the case of infectious diseases, partly because it is the method of macrophags to absorb the contents of the higher cells extremely slowly. The mode of action is well seen in the atrophy of an egg-cell (Fig. 8), where the surrounding macrophags gradually seize hold of the granules within it and carry these off. As the process goes on, the ovum becomes reduced to a shapeless mass, and finally leaves only a few fragments, or disappears completely. M. Matchinsky[1] has studied the series of events in my laboratory, and I am myself well assured of the importance of the action of macrophags in the atrophy of the ovary.

The phenomena of atrophy in general and of senile decay afford other cases of tissue destruction in which the phago-

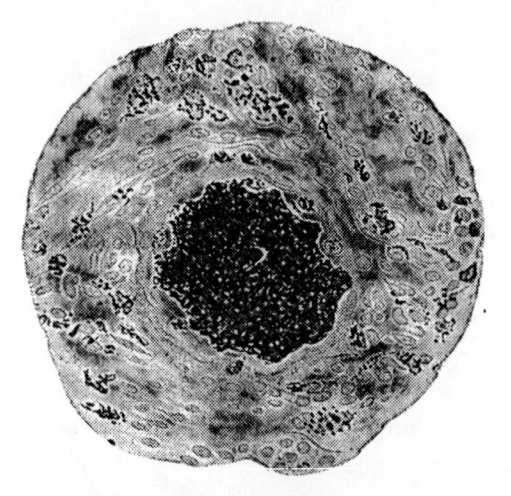

FIG. 8.—Ovum of a Bitch in process of destruction by Phagocytes, which are full of fatty granules.
(After M. Matchinsky.)

cytic character of the process is more modified and obscure than in nerve-cells and ova.

It is well known that progressive muscular debility is an accompaniment of old age. Physical work is seldom given to men over sixty years of age, as it is notorious that they are less capable of it. Their muscular movements are feebler and soon bring on fatigue; their actions are slow and painful. Even old men whose mental vigour is unimpaired admit their muscular weakness. The physical

[1] *Annales de l'Institut Pasteur*, 1900, vol. xiv. p. 113.

correlate of this condition is an actual atrophy of the muscles, and has for long been known to observers. More than half a century ago, Kölliker,[1] one of the founders of histology, devoted some attention to this matter, and described the senile modification of muscular tissue in the following words:—" In old age there is a true atrophy of the muscles. The fibres are much more slender; there are deposited in their substance numerous yellow or brown granules and many globular nuclei. These nuclei are frequently arranged in longitudinal series and present such signs of active division as are found in embryonic tissue."

Other investigators afterwards made similar observations. Vulpian[2] and Douaud[3] have stated that a multiplication of nuclei takes places in the atrophying muscles of the old.

As the senile degeneration of muscular tissue appeared to be important in my study of the mechanism of senescence, M. Weinberg and I examined several cases of muscular atrophy in old human beings and lower animals. We were able to recognise the phenomena observed by our predecessors. In senile atrophy the muscular fibres contain many nuclei, and these, increasing rapidly, bring about an almost complete disappearance of the contractile substance (Fig. 9). The fibres preserve their striation for a certain time but eventually lose it and appear to contain an amorphous mass with numerous, rapidly multiplying nuclei.

The investigators who had recorded these facts thought of them only as curious. It is plain, in the first place, however, that this remarkable and rapid multiplication is a proof that senile atrophy is not due to failure of cell pro-

---

[1] *Eléments d'histologie humaine*, French translation, 1856, p. 222.
[2] *Leçons sur la physiologie du système nerveux*, 1866.
[3] *De la dégénérescence graisseuse des muscles chez des vieillards.* Paris, 1867.

liferation, although the latter has frequently been suggested as the mechanism of senescence. In muscular atrophy, cell-multiplication, so far from failing, greatly increases. We may add muscular atrophy to the blanching of hair and the decay of nerve-cells as another instance showing that senile degeneration is not the result of cells ceasing to be able to

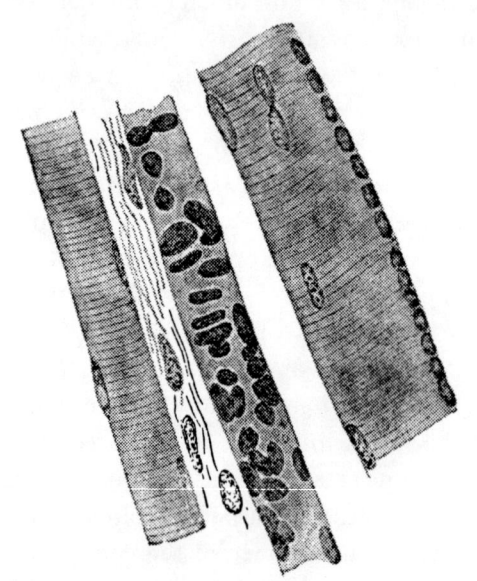

FIG. 9.—Degeneration of striated muscle Fibres from the auricular muscle of a man aged 87 years.
(From a preparation made by Dr. Weinberg.)

multiply. Just as in the atrophy of the brain there is an increase in the volume of neurogloea, the substance in which the neuronophags are found, so also in the atrophy of the muscles there is an increase of muscular nuclei. Along with the increase of nuclei, however, there is an increase of the protoplasmic substance of the fibres known as sarcoplasm. The latter replaces the myoplasm, the specific striated substance of muscles, by a process which must be regarded as parallel with phagocytosis. In a normal muscle the two substances and the sarcoplasmic nuclei are in equilibrium, but in old age the sarcoplasm and its nuclei increase at the expense of the myoplasm. The equilibrium is destroyed with the result that the muscular power is weakened. In these conditions the sarcoplasm acts phagocytically with regard to the myoplasm, just as the chromophag becomes the phagocyte of the pigment of the hair, or the neuronophag devours the nerve-cell.

The investigation of other cases of muscular atrophy, as, for instance, that of the caudal muscles of frog-tadpoles, confirms the significance of the process that I have observed in old age. In the two cases, what takes place is the destruction of the contractile material of the muscles by myophags, a special kind of phagocyte.

It is one of the curiosities of senile atrophy that whilst there is hardening or sclerosis of so many organs, the skeleton, the most solid part of our frame-work, becomes less dense, so that the bones are friable, the condition often leading to serious accidents in old people. The bones become porous, and lose weight. It is difficult to believe that macrophags, although they destroy softer elements such as nerve-cells or muscle fibres, can be able to gnaw through a hard material like bone impregnated with mineral salts. As a matter of fact, the mechanism of bone atrophy must be placed in a different category from the phagocytosis of other organs. It is brought about, however, by the agency of cells very like some of the macrophags. These cells contain many nuclei, and are known as osteoclasts. They form round about the bony lamellæ and lead to their destruction, but are incapable of breaking off fragments of bone and dissolving them in their interiors. Although the intimate mechanism of this destructive action is not thoroughly understood, it seems probable that the cells secrete some acid which softens bone by dissolving the lime salts. The process can be observed in the different varieties of caries of the bone, and in the bony atrophy of old age as is represented in Fig. 10.

By the action of the osteoclasts, which themselves are macrophags, part of the lime in the skeleton is dissolved during old age and passes into the general circulation. This is probably a source of the lime which is deposited so readily in the different tissues of old people. Whilst the bones become lighter, the cartilages become bony, the inter-

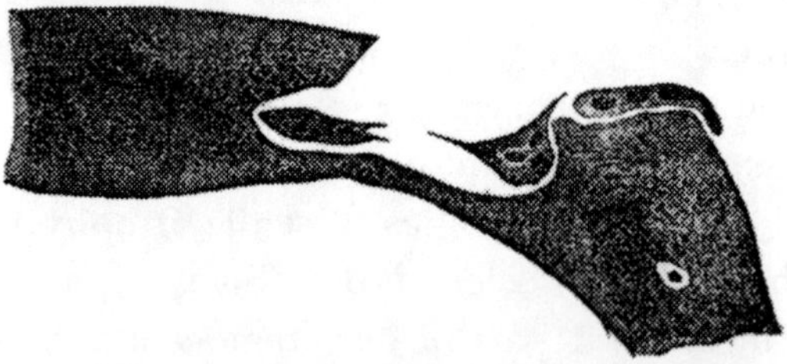

FIG. 10.—Destruction by osteoclasts of bony matter in the sternum of a man aged 81 years.
(From a preparation made by Dr. Weinberg.)

vertebrate discs in particular becoming impregnated with salts, so that the well-known senile malformation of the backbone is produced.

As a result of this displacement of lime in old age, the blood-vessels become modified in a distinctive fashion. Atheroma of the arteries is not invariable in old people, but it occurs extremely frequently. In this form of degeneration, lime salts are deposited in the walls of the cells, so that they become hard and friable. Several others, among whom I may mention Durand-Fardel and Sauvage, have laid stress on the coincidence of atheromatous lesions of the arteries and senile degeneration of the bones. The relations between the two alterations are very evident in the skull; the meningeal artery becomes sinuous and atheromatous, and the grooves on the inner side of the bones of the skull in which it runs, flatten out, and become larger because of other malformations.[1]

There is no disharmony in the nature of old people so striking as this transference of the lime salts from the skeleton to the blood-vessels, producing as it does a dangerous softening of the former, and a hardening of the latter that interferes with their function of carrying nutrition to the organs. It is the manifestation of an extraordinary disturbance of the properties of the cells that compose the body. The atheromatous condition of the arteries is closely linked with arterial sclerosis, an affection which is very common, although not constant, in the aged. The whole question of these vascular alterations is extremely complex, and before it can be cleared up, a number of special investigations must be made.

Probably diseases of the arteries of different kinds, and arising from different causes, are grouped under the terms atheroma and sclerosis. In some cases the lesions are inflammatory and are due to the poisons of microbes. An example of such an origin is the case of syphilitic sclerosis, in which the specific microbes (spirilla of Schaudinn) lead to precocious senescence. In other cases the arteries show phenomena of degeneration resulting in the formation of calcareous platelets which interfere with the circulation of the blood.

Investigations which have been made in recent years have led to very interesting results concerning the origin of atheroma of the arteries. In most cases, attempts to produce such lesions of the arteries by experimental

[1] Demange, *Étude sur la vieillesse*, 1886, p. 118.

methods have not succeeded, but M. Josué[1] has been able to produce true arterial atheroma in rabbits by injecting into them adrenaline, the secretion of the suprarenal capsules.

This experiment has been repeated many times and is now well known. Later on, M. Boveri[2] obtained a similar result by injecting nicotine, the poison of tobacco. It is obvious, therefore, that amongst the arterial diseases which play so great a part in senescence, some are chronic inflammations produced by microbes, whilst others are brought about by poisons introduced from without.

It is easy to understand, therefore, why these diseases of the arteries are not always present in old age, although they are very common.

The part played by the secretion of the suprarenal glands in the production of arterial disease has brought renewed attention to a theory which supposed that certain glandular organs in the body play a preponderating part in senile degeneration. Dr. Lorand[3] in particular has argued that "senility is a morbid process due to the degeneration of the thyroid gland and of other ductless glands which normally regulate the nutrition of the body." It has long been noticed that persons affected with myxodema, as a result of the degeneration of the thyroid gland, look like very old people. Everyone who has seen the cretins in Savoy, Switzerland, or the Tyrol, must have noticed the aged appearance of these victims, although very often they are quite young. The condition of cretinism, with its profound bodily changes, is the result of degeneration of the thyroid gland. On the other hand, it is well known that

[1] *C. R. de la Société de Biologie*, 14 November, 1903.
[2] *Clinica medica*, 1905, *n.* 6.
[3] *Bulletins de la Société royale des sciences-medicales de Bruxelles*, 1905, *n.* 4, p. 105.

in old people the thyroid and the suprarenals frequently show cystic degeneration. It is quite probable, therefore, that these so-called vascular glands have their share in producing senility. Many facts show that they destroy certain poisons which have entered the body, and it is easy to see that, if they have become functionless, the tissues are threatened with poisoning. It does not follow, however, that their action in producing senility is exclusive, or even preponderating. M. Weinberg, at the Pasteur Institute, made special investigations on this point, and found that the thyroid gland and the suprarenal capsules were almost invariably normal in old animals (cat, dog, horse), although the latter showed unmistakable signs of senility. Similarly in an old man of 80 years, who died from pneumonia, the thyroid gland was quite normal.

It must not be forgotten that the aged very often die from infectious diseases such as pneumonia, tuberculosis, and erysipelas. In these diseases the vascular glands generally, and the thyroid gland in particular, are very often affected, with the result that what is due to infection has been set down as a symptom of old age.[1]

Although the appearance of patients from whom the thyroid gland has been removed, or in whom it has degenerated spontaneously, recalls that of old people, it is possible to exaggerate the similarity. In the masterly accounts of such unfortunates, recently compiled by the well-known surgeon Kocher[2] there are many points which are characteristic, without being typical, of old people.

Oedema of the skin which characterises thyroid patients

[1] Sarbach, *Mittheilungen a. d. Grenzgeb. d. Med. u. Chir.*, vol. xv. 1906.
[2] *Verhandlungen d. Kongr. f. innere Medicin.* Wiesbaden, 1906, pp. 59, 98.

is by no means usual in old age. The loss of hair, normal in the patients, is not a character of old age. In myxedematous women, menstruation is very active; it ceases in old women. The great muscular development of myxedematous patients distinguishes them from old people.

Physiological investigation does not support the existence of any strong affinity between old age and affection of the thyroid gland. It is known that removal of the thyroid is followed by cachexia only in young subjects, MM. Bourneville and Bricon[1] having shown that the tendency to cachexia after extirpation of the thyroid ceases almost abruptly at the age of thirty. That age may be taken as the limit of youth, of the time when growth is vigorous and the function of the thyroid most active. Cases of cachexia, where the thyroid gland has been removed in old persons from fifty to seventy, are very rare.

Rodents (rats, rabbits) support the removal of the thyroid extremely well, without signs of cachexia, although these are normally short-lived creatures. According to Horsley[2] extirpation of the thyroid is not followed by cachexia in birds or rodents and is followed by it only very slowly in ruminants and horses; it produces the condition invariably but slightly in man and monkeys and extremely seriously in carnivora. If this series be compared with the information given in the next section of this volume on the relative ages which the animals in question attain, it will be seen that there is no correspondence.

In short, whilst I do not deny that the vascular glands may take a share in the causation of senility, in so far as

[1] *Archives de Neurologie*, 1886.
[2] Die Function d. Schilddrüse, *Virchow's Festschrift*, vol. i. 1891, p. 369.

they are destroyers of poisons, I cannot agree with the theory of Dr. Lorand.

I think it indubitable that in senescence the most active factor is some alteration in the higher cells of the body, accompanied by a destruction of these by macrophags which gradually usurp the places of the higher elements and replace them by fibrous tissue. Such a process affects the organs of secretion (kidneys), the reproductive organs, and in a modified form the skin, the mucous membranes, and the skeleton. The testes are amongst the organs which resist invasion by macrophags. I have already given an example ("The Nature of Man," p. 98) of an old man of 94 in whom active spermatozoa were produced. I know of a similar case, the age being 103 years. Such cases are not rare, and not only in old men, but in old animals, the testes continue to be active. Dr. Weinberg and I have investigated these organs in a dog which died at the age of 22 years after several years of pronounced senility. Many of the organs of the animal exhibited serious invasions by macrophags but the testes were extremely active, the cells being in free proliferation and producing abundant spermatozoa (Fig. 11). In harmony with this condition of the sexual organs, the sexual instincts of the animal remained normal. We have investigated another dog which died at the age of eighteen years. In this case the testes were cancerous and there was no possibility of the production of spermatozoa. None the less, this dog although markedly

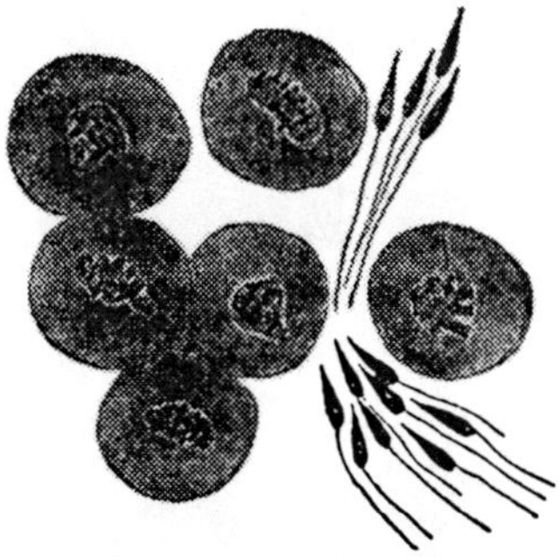

FIG. 11.—Testis tissue from a dog aged twenty-two years. (From a preparation made by Dr. Weinberg.)

senile (Fig. 12) still showed sexual instincts until shortly before it died.

It is manifest that the tissues do not invariably degenerate in old age, nor do all the organs that are modified in old age show destruction by phagocytes and replacement by connective tissue. Organs which produce phagocytes, such as the spleen, the spinal marrow and the lymphatic glands, certainly show traces in old age of fibrous degenera-

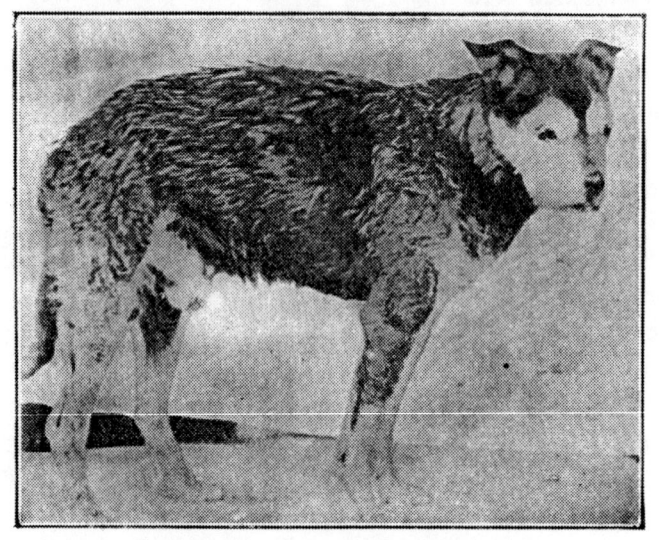

Fig. 12.—An old dog, aged eighteen years.

tion but remain sufficiently active to produce macrophags which destroy the higher cellular elements of the body. I have frequently noticed cell division in such organs, and as an example may give the case of the bone marrow taken from a man of 81 years (Fig. 13).

The eye is an organ that is modified in old age without the action of macrophags. Cataract and the senile arc which appears as a milky ring at the edge of the cornea

MECHANISM OF SENILITY

are frequent in old age. These modifications are due to impregnation of the parts affected by fatty matter which makes them opaque. This deposition of fat[1] has been attributed to defective nutrition. In most organs such fatty degeneration is followed by phagocytosis, but the cornea and the crystalline lens are exempt from this consequence for anatomical reasons. Most organs possess in addition to their higher elements a constant source of macrophags. Such a source of phagocytosis is the neurogloea in nervous tissues, the sarcoplasm in muscular tissues; the bones contain osteoclasts and the liver and the kidneys are readily invaded by phagocytes from the blood. The lens and the cornea have no cells that are able to become macrophags.

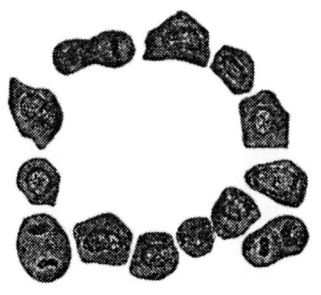

FIG. 13.—Bone marrow from the sternum of a man aged eighty-one years. (From a preparation made by Dr. Weinberg.)

Some infectious diseases bring about precocious senility. A syphilitic child is "a miniature old man, with wrinkled face, skin dull and discoloured and flabby and hanging in folds as if it were too large."[2] In such a case the active agent is the microbe of syphilis which has poisoned the child on the breast of its mother. It is no mere analogy to suppose that human senescence is the result of a slow but chronic poisoning of the organism. Such poisons, if not completely destroyed or eliminated, weaken the tissues, the functions of which become altered or enfeebled, so that,

[1] Fuss, Der Greisenbogen, in *Virchow's Archiv*, 1905, vol. clxxxii. p. 407; S. Toufesco, *Sur le cristallin*, Paris, 1906.

[2] Edmond Fournier, *Stigmates dystrophiques de l'hérédosyphilis*, Paris, 1898, p. 4.

amongst other changes, there is deposition of fatty matter. The phagocytes resist the influence of invading poisons better than any of the other cells of the body and sometimes are stimulated by them. The general result of such conditions is that there comes to be a struggle between the higher cells and the phagocytes in which the latter have the advantage.

The answer to the question as to whether our senescence can be ameliorated must be approached from several points of view. This course I shall now follow.

PART II

LONGEVITY IN THE ANIMAL KINGDOM

I

THEORIES OF LONGEVITY

Relation between longevity and size—Longevity and the period of growth—Longevity and the doubling in weight after birth—Longevity and rate of reproduction—Probable relation between longevity and the nature of the food

THE duration of the life of animals varies within very wide limits. Some, as for instance, the males of certain wheel animalculæ (Rotifera) complete their cycle of life from birth to death in 50 or 60 hours, whilst others, like some reptiles, live more than 100 years, and quite possibly may live for two or three centuries.

Enquiry has been made for many years as to whether there are laws governing these different durations of life. Even the most casual observation of domesticated animals has shown that, as a general rule, small animals do not live so long as large ones; mice, guinea pigs, and rabbits for instance, have shorter lives than geese, ducks, and sheep, whilst these again are survived by horses, deer, and camels. Of all the mammals which have lived under the protection of man, the elephant is at once the largest, and the most long-lived.

However, it is not difficult to show that there is no absolute relation between size and longevity, since parrots, ravens, and geese live much longer than many mammals, and than some much larger birds.

As a general rule it may be said that a large animal takes more time than a small one to reach maturity, and it has been inferred from this that the length of the periods of gestation and of growth were in proportion to the longevity. Buffon[1] long ago stated his opinion that the "total duration of life bore some definite relation to the length of the period of growth." Therefore, as the period of growth is, so to say, inherent in the species, longevity would have to be regarded as a very stable phenomenon. Just as any species has acquired a fixed and practically invariable size, so it would have acquired a definite longevity. Buffon, therefore, thought that the duration of life did not depend on habits or mode of life, or on the nature of food, that, in fact, nothing could change its rigid laws, except an excess of nourishment.

Taking as his standard the total period of development of the body, Buffon came to the conclusion that the duration of life is six or seven times that of the period of growth. Man, for instance, he said, who takes 14 years to grow, can live 6 or 7 times that period, that is to say, 90 or 100 years. The horse, which reaches its full size in 4 years, can live 6 or 7 times that length of time, that is to say from 25 to 30 years. The stag takes 5 or 6 years to grow, and reckoned in the same way, its longevity should be 35 to 40 years.

Flourens[2] although supporting his principle, thought that Buffon had been inexact in calculating the period of growth. In his opinion a better result can be obtained by taking the limit of growth as that age at which the epiphyses of the long bones unite with the bones them-

[1] *Histoire naturelle générale et particulière*, vol. ii. Paris, 1749.
[2] *De la longévité humaine et de la quantité de vie sur le globe*, Paris, 1855.

THEORIES OF LONGEVITY

selves. Using such a mode of computation, Flourens laid down that an animal lived 5 times the length of its period of growth. Man, for instance, takes 20 years to grow, and he can live for 5 times that space, that is to say, 100 years; the camel takes 8 to grow, and lives 5 times as long, *i.e.*, 40 years; the horse, 5 to grow, and lives 25 years.

However, even if we consider only the mammalia, it is impossible to accept Flourens' law, without considerable reserve. Weismann [1] has referred to the case of the horse, which is completely adult at 4, but lives not merely 5 times that period, but 10 or even 12 times. Mice grow extremely quickly, so that they are able to reproduce at the age of 4 months. Even if we take 6 months as their period of growth, their longevity of 5 years is twice as long as it would be according to the rule of Flourens. Amongst domesticated animals, the sheep is slow in reaching maturity; it does not acquire its adult set of teeth until it is 5 years old, and cannot be regarded as adult until then. None the less, at the age of 8 or 10 years, it loses its teeth and begins to grow old, whilst by 14 it is quite senile.[2] The longevity of the sheep, therefore, is not quite three times its period of growth.

If we turn to other vertebrates, the variations in the relation of growth and the duration of life are still greater. Parrots, for instance, the longevity of which is extremely great, grow very quickly. At the age of 2 years, they have acquired the adult plumage and are able to reproduce, whilst the smaller species are in the same condition at the age of one. Incubation, moreover, is very short, not more than 25 days, and in some species not three weeks. None the less, parrots are birds which enjoy a

[1] *Ueber die Dauer des Lebens*, Jena, 1882, p. 4.
[2] Brehm, *La vie des animaux, Mammifères*, vol. ii. p. 623.

quite remarkable longevity. The incubation period of domestic geese is 30 days, and their period of growth is also short. However, they may reach a great age, cases of 80 years and of 100 years being on record. In contrast with these, ostriches, the incubation period of which is 42 to 49 days, and which take 3 years to become adult, have a relatively short life.

H. Milne-Edwards[1] many years ago contended that there was no importance in the supposed law of relation between gestation and longevity. He sums up his criticism as follows: "Although the period of uterine life is longer in the horse, that animal does not live so long as a human being; and some birds, the incubation of which only lasts a few weeks, can live more than a century."

Bunge[2] has recently taken up the study of the relations between the duration of growth and longevity, and has suggested a new means of investigation. He has observed that the period in which the new-born mammal doubles its weight is a good index of the rapidity of its growth. He has shown that whilst a human child requires 180 days to reach double its weight at birth, the horse, the longevity of which is very much less, doubles its weight in 60 days; a calf takes only 47 days for this; a kid 15 days; a pig 14 days; a cat $9\frac{1}{2}$; and a dog only 9 days. Although these facts are very interesting, the exceptions are too great to make it possible to base a law of longevity upon them. The period of weight-doubling in the horse is nearly 7 times longer than that in the dog, and yet the longevity of the horse is not more than 3 times that of the dog. The goat, which takes much longer than the dog to double its weight, has a shorter total life.

[1] *Leçons sur la physiologie et l'anatomie comparée*, vol. ix. 1870, p. 446.
[2] *Archiv f. die gesammte Physiologie*, Bonn, 1903, vol. xcv. p. 606.

I observed myself that new-born mice quadruple their weight in the first 24 hours. The doubling of weight in their case requires a time 36 times less long than that of the cat, and yet the cat lives only 5 times as long as the mouse.

It is fair to say, however, that Bunge himself does not draw a definite conclusion from these figures and has published them only to stimulate interest in the subject. He is against the view of Flourens, and points out that although the multiple 5 is valid for man, it is not so in the case of the horse which finishes its growth in 4 years and yet reaches the age of 40 much less often than human beings attain that of 100 years.

Although it is impossible to admit the existence of exact relations between size and the period of growth on the one side, and longevity on the other, in the mode which Buffon and Flourens have followed, it is none the less true that there is something intrinsic in each kind of animal which sets a definite limit to the length of years it can attain. The purely physiological conditions which determine this limit leave room for a considerable amount of variation in longevity. Duration of life therefore, is a character which can be influenced by the environment. Weismann in his well-known essay on the duration of life, has laid stress on this side of the problem. Longevity, according to him, although in the last resort depending on the physiological properties of the cells of which the organism is composed, can be adapted to the conditions of existence and influenced by natural selection, like other characters useful for the existence of the species.

If a species is to remain in existence, its members must be able to reproduce and the progeny must be able to reach adult life so that they in their turn may reproduce. Now, it happens that there are some animals the fecundity of which is extremely limited. Most birds which are adapted to aerial life, and the weight of which is therefore to be kept down, lay very few eggs. This happens in the case of birds of prey, such as eagles and vultures. These birds nest only once a year, and generally rear two or frequently only a single nestling. In such circumstances the duration of life becomes a factor in the preservation of the species, more important since eggs and chicks are subject to many dangers. Eggs are devoured by many kinds of animals, whilst unseasonable cold may kill the chicks. If the members of such a species were incapable of living long, the unfavourable conditions of life would soon lead to extinction. Those animals which reproduce rapidly generally have a relatively brief duration of life. Mice, rats, rabbits, and many other rodents seldom live more than 5 or 10 years, but reproduce with enormous rapidity. It is almost possible to imagine that there is some sort of intimate link, possibly physiological, between longevity and low fertility. It is a current opinion that reproduction wastes the maternal organism and that mothers of many children grow old prematurely and seldom reach an advanced age. This would seem to mean that fecundity was the cause of the short duration of life. However, we must guard ourselves against such a theory. Longevity, at least in the case of vertebrate animals, differs extremely little in the two sexes, although the cost of the new generation to the adult organism is very much greater in the case of the female than of the male parent. None the less, females frequently reach a great age, especially in the human race where women reach 100 years, or live beyond that time, much more often than men.

Low fertility, however, cannot itself be regarded as a cause of longevity, as there are some very fertile animals

THEORIES OF LONGEVITY

which none the less attain great ages. There are parrots which lay two or three times a year, producing six to nine eggs in each clutch. The ducks (Anatidæ) are distinguished for considerable longevity and very high fertility, each nest containing rarely less than six and sometimes as many as sixteen eggs. The common Sheldrake lays from twenty to thirty eggs. Tame ducks, in some parts of the tropics, lay an egg daily throughout the season. Wild ducks lay from seven to fourteen eggs in one nest. Ducks and geese, none the less, frequently attain considerable ages, ducks having been known to live for 29 years. Even the common fowl, which is a notoriously prolific bird, may reach an age of twenty to thirty years.

It will be said, however, that these birds are exposed to many enemies during youth. Chickens, ducklings, and goslings are ready prey for hawks, foxes and small carnivora. The longevity is possibly to be explained as an adaptation for the preservation of the species by compensating for the great destruction of the young. Weismann explains in this way the longevity of many aquatic birds and other creatures that are much preyed on. It must be noted, however, that the longevity cannot depend on the risks run by the young birds, but must have arisen independently. If this had not occurred, creatures, the young of which are destroyed in great numbers, would have ceased to exist, as many species have disappeared in geological time. The longevity of prolific animals, the young of which are destroyed in numbers, must be due to some cause which is neither fertility nor the destruction of their offspring. This cause must be sought in the physiological processes of the organism and can be attributed neither to the length of the period of growth nor to the size attained by the adults.

After having discussed various theories of the cause of the duration of life, M. Oustalet,[1] in a most interesting essay on the longevity of vertebrates, came to the conclusion that diet was the chief factor. He thinks that there is a "definite relation between diet and longevity. For the most part herbivorous animals live longer than carnivorous forms, probably because the former find their food with ease and regularity, whilst the latter alternate between semi-starvation and repletion." There are certainly many instances which give support to the view. Elephants and parrots, for instance, are vegetarian and reach very great ages. On the other hand, there exist long-living carnivorous animals. Many observations have made it certain that owls and eagles reach great ages, and these birds live on animal food. Ravens, which live on carrion, are also notorious for the duration of their lives. There is no exact knowledge as to the ages reached by crocodiles, but although these live on flesh, it is certain that their longevity is great.

We must seek elsewhere for the real factors that control duration of life. Before stating my conclusion, I will review what is known as to the duration of life of different animals.

[1] *La Nature*, May 12, 1900, p. 378.

II.

LONGEVITY IN THE ANIMAL KINGDOM

> Longevity in the lower animals—Instances of long life in sea-anemones and other invertebrates—Duration of life of insects—Duration of life of " cold-blooded " vertebrates—Duration of life of birds—Duration of life of mammals—Inequality of the duration of life in males and females—Relations between longevity and fertility of the organism

It is wonderful to what an extent the duration of life varies amongst animals, the slightest examination of the facts showing that very many factors must be involved.

As the higher animals are nearly always larger than invertebrates, if there be a definite relation between longevity and size, one would expect to find that vertebrates live longer than invertebrates. However, this is not the case. Amongst animals of extremely simple organisation, there are some which reach a great age. A striking example of this is found in sea-anemones. These animals have a very simple structure, without a separate digestive canal, and with a badly developed, diffused nervous system, and yet have lived very long in captivity. More than forty years ago, I remember having seen in the possession of M. Lloyd, the Director of the Aquarium at Hamburg, an anemone that he had kept alive for several dozen years in a glass bowl. Another sea-anemone, belonging to the species *Actinia mesembryanthemum*, is known to have lived 66 years. It was captured in 1828 by Dalyell, a

Scottish zoologist, and was then quite adult, and probably about 7 years old. It survived its owner for 36 years, and died in Edinburgh in 1887, the cause of death being unknown. Although they are thus capable of living so long, the rate of growth of members of this species is rapid, and their fertility is very high. According to Dalyell, these anemones reach the adult condition in 15 months. The specimen in his possession, in the 20 years from 1828 to 1848 produced 334 larvæ, then after a period of sterility it gave birth, in one night (1857) to 230 young anemones. This extraordinary prolificness decreased with age, but even when it was 58 years old it used to produce from 5 to 20 at a time. In the seven years from 1872 onwards, it gave birth to 150 young anemones.[1] This animal, which certainly was not more than the fortieth or the fiftieth of the weight of an adult rabbit, lived six or seven times as long.

Ashworth and Nelson Annandale have published their observations on another sea-anemone, of the species *Sagartia troglodytes*, which was 50 years old. It differed from younger examples only in being less prolific.

There are other polyps, such as *Flabellum*, which do not live more than 24 years, although we have no knowledge as to the cause of the different duration of life.

The variation in the length of the life of molluscs and insects is extremely great. Some species of gasteropods (*Vitrina, Succinea*) live only a very few years, whilst others (*Natica heros*) can reach thirty years. Some of the marine bivalves, as for instance, *Tridacna gigas*, can live to sixty or a hundred years.[2]

Insects are animals as variable in their duration of life as they are in other respects. Some live only a few weeks;

[1] Ashworth and Annandale, *Proceedings of the R. Society of Edinburgh*, vol. xxv. part iv. 1904.
[2] *Bronn's Klassen u. Ordnungen des Thierreichs*, vol. iii. p. 466.

LONGEVITY IN THE ANIMAL KINGDOM

some of the plant-lice, for instance, die in a month. In the same order of Insects, however, (Hemiptera) there are species of cicada which live thirteen to seventeen years, that is to say, much longer than such little Rodents as rats, mice, and guinea-pigs. The larva of an American species spends seventeen years buried in the ground in orchards, where it feeds on the roots of apple trees, and the species is known as *Cicada septemdecim,* because of this duration of life. In the adult stage the insect lives little more than a month, just time enough to lay the eggs, and bring into the world the new generation, which in its turn will not appear above ground until after another period of seventeen years.

Between these extremes of long and short life, there is to be found amongst insects almost every gradation of longevity. Science, in its present state, has failed to find any law governing these facts. Rules which hold good up to a certain point in the case of the higher animals break down in their application to insects. The large grasshoppers and locusts, for instance, live a much shorter time than many minute beetles. Queen bees, the fertility of which is very great, live two or three years and may reach a fifth year, whilst worker bees, which are infertile, die in the first year of their existence. Female ants, although these are small and extremely prolific, reach the age of seven years.[1]

We know so little about the physiological processes of insects, that we cannot as yet make even a guess at the cause of this great variation in their longevity. It is more probable that we shall find some explanation in the case of vertebrates concerning which we know much more.

Analysis of the facts shows that whilst in the evolution

[1] Weismann, *The Duration of Life,* in "Essays on Heredity" (English translation), Oxford, 1889.

from fish to mammal there has been a great increase in complexity of organisation, there has at the same time been a reduction in the duration of life. As a general rule, it may be laid down that the lower vertebrates live longer than mammals.

The facts about the longevity of fish are not very numerous, but it seems clear that these animals reach a great age. The ancient Romans, who used to keep eels in aquaria, have noted that these fish would live for more than sixty years. There is reason to believe that salmon can live for a century, whilst pike live much longer. There is, for instance, the much quoted instance of the pike stated by Gessner to have been captured in 1230 and to have lived for 267 years afterwards. Carps are regarded as equally long lived, Buffon setting down their period of life as 150 years. There is a popular idea that the carp in the lakes at Fontainebleau and Chantilly are several centuries old, but E. Blanchard throws doubt on the accuracy of this estimate, inasmuch as during revolutionary times most of the carp were eaten when the palaces were overrun by the populace. There is no doubt, however, that the life of carp may be very long indeed. Not very much is known about the duration of life in batrachians, but it is certain at least that some small frogs may live twelve or sixteen years, and toads as many as thirty-six years.

More is known about the life of reptiles. Crocodiles and caymans, which are large and which grow very slowly, attain great ages. In the Paris Museum of Natural History there are crocodiles which have been kept for more than forty years without showing signs of senescence. Turtles, although they are smaller than crocodiles, live still longer. A tortoise has lived for eighty years in the garden of the Governor of Cape Town, and is believed to have reached the age of two hundred years. Another tortoise, a native of the Galapagos Islands, is known to be 175 years old, whilst a specimen in the London Zoological Gardens is 150 years old. A land tortoise (*Testudo marginata*) has been kept in Norfolk, England, for a century. I am informed that in the Archbishop's palace at Canterbury, there is to be seen the carapace of a tortoise which was brought to the Palace in 1623 and which lived there for 107 years.[1] Another tortoise, brought to Fulham by Archbishop Laud, lived in the Palace for 128 years. I have already referred to a specimen of *Testudo mauritanica*, the history of which is known for 86 years, but which is probably much older.

Very little is known as to the longevity of lizards and serpents, but it may be inferred from what I have said about other reptiles that reptiles as a class are able to reach great ages.

It is an easy inference that the great duration of life in cold-blooded animals is associated with the slowness of the physiological processes in these creatures. The circulation, for instance, is so slow, that the heart of a tortoise beats only 20 to 25 times in a minute. Weismann has suggested that one of the factors influencing the duration of life is the rapidity or slowness of the vital activities, the times taken by the processes of absorption and nutrition.

On the other hand, the blood is hot and the vital activities are rapid in birds, and yet birds may attain great ages. Although in the last chapter I gave a number of examples, the subject is so important that I propose to go further into details. The possibility of this is due to an admirable set of details brought together by Mr. J. H. Gurney.[2] In his

---

[1] Oustalet, "*La Longévité chez les Animaux vertébrés,*" *La Nature*, May 12, 1900, p. 378.

[2] "*On the Comparative Ages to which Birds live,*" *The Ibis*, Jan., 1899, vol. v. p. 19.

list, in which are included more than fifty species of birds, the lowest figures are from eight and a half to nine years (*Podargus cuvieri, Chelidon urbica*), and a duration of life so short is an exception, a period of from fifteen to twenty years being more common. Canaries have lived in captivity from 17 to 20 years, and goldfinches up to 23 years. Field larks have lived for 24 years, the Lesser Black-backed Gull 31 years and the Herring Gull 44 years. Birds of medium size may live for several dozens of years, whether they live on animal or on vegetable food, whether they are prolific or lay very few eggs. I will quote only a few instances. Of forty parrots the minimum and maximum ages were respectively 15 and 81 years, and the average 43 years. Without accepting the truth of the story mentioned by Humboldt according to which certain parrots survived an extinct race of Indians, at least we may be certain that great ages have sometimes been reached by these birds. Levaillant mentions a parrot (*Psittacus erithaceus*) which lost its memory at the age of 60 years, its sight at 90 years, and which died aged 93 years. Another individual, probably of the same species, is reported by J. Jennings to have reached the age of 77. Jones, Layard, and Butler are the authorities for instances of Sulphur-crested Cockatoos having reached respectively 30, 72 and 81 years. M. Abrahams states that an Amazon (*Chrysotis amazonica*) lived 102 years. I myself have observed two cases of great longevity in the same species of parrot. One of these birds died at the age of 82 years, apparently simply from old age, whilst the other, which was in my possession for several years before it died at the age of 70 to 75 years, was vigorous, showing no signs of senility, but died of pneumonia.

Mr. Gurney found that parrots were not the only birds

capable of reaching a great age. One raven reached 69 years and another 50, an Eagle-owl (*Bubo maximus*) 68 years, another 53, a condor 52, an imperial eagle 56, a common heron 60, a wild goose 80, and a common swan 70 years. None of these examples approaches the legendary three centuries attributed to the swan, but it is evident that many different kinds of birds may attain great age. I can add some cases to those of Mr. Gurney. In the Royal Park at Schönbrunn, near Vienna, a white-headed vulture (*Neophron percnopterus*) died aged 118 years, a golden eagle (*Aquila chrysaëtus*) aged 104, and another aged 80 (according to Oustalet). Mr. Pycraft (*Country Life*, June 25th, 1904) reported that a female eagle, captured in Norway in 1829, had been brought to England and had lived for 75 years. In the last thirty years of its life, it had produced ninety eggs. The same writer mentions the case of a falcon having lived to 162 years.

The collection of facts that I have passed in review make it manifest that birds may have a great duration of life, but that reptiles surpass them in this respect. Birds certainly do not reach the very great ages of crocodiles and tortoises.

Longevity, therefore, is reduced as we ascend in the scale of vertebrate life. We find a still greater reduction when we turn from birds to mammals. Some mammals, it is true, may live as long as birds. Elephants are a good instance. It used to be thought that these giant mammals could live three or four centuries, but I can find no confirmation of the legend, which seems as mythical as that relating to the life of swans. There are no exact data as to the ages reached by wild elephants, but it has been stated that in captivity an elephant rarely but occasionally has completed its century. In zoological gardens and in good menageries, where elephants are well cared for, they seldom live more than 20 to 25 years. Chevrette, an African elephant presented to the Jardin des Plantes by Mehemet Ali, in 1825, lived for only 30 years. In the official list of the Indian Government, which gives the deaths of elephants, it appears that of 138 examples, only one lived more than 20 years after it had been purchased (Brehm's *Mammals*).

Flourens, using his own formula, assigned the age of 150 years to elephants as their epiphyses do not fuse with the long bones until the age of 30. So far, I know of no fact to support the conclusion, although it seems fairly well established that occasionally an elephant may reach a century. It is stated that one elephant was in service throughout the whole period of more than 140 years in which Ceylon was occupied by the Dutch. This elephant was found in the stables in 1656. Natives with special knowledge of elephants set down their duration of life as from 80 to 150 years, but say that they begin to grow old at from 50 to 60 years of age. My general conclusion from the facts is that the life of these very large mammals is about the same as that of man who is very much smaller.

Centenarians, extremely rare amongst elephants, do not appear to exist in any other kind of mammals except man. The rhinoceros, another large mammal which is a native of the same countries as the elephant, does not reach a great age. According to Oustalet an Indian rhinoceros died in the menagerie of the Paris Museum at about the age of 25 years, and showed all the signs of senility. Another Indian rhinoceros lived for 37 years in the London Zoological Gardens. Grindon has stated his opinion that the rhinoceros may live for 70 or 80 years, but this seems rather an inference from the slowness of growth than a statement of observed fact.

Horses and cattle are large animals, but do not enjoy very long lives. The usual duration of life in horses is from 15 to 30 years. They begin to grow old about 10 years, and in very rare cases may reach 40 or more. A Welsh pony is said to have reached the age of sixty, but such a case is excessively rare. Two other extreme cases are that of a horse belonging to the Bishop of Metz which died at the age of 50 years, and the charger of Field-Marshal Lacy which died at 46.

The duration of life of cattle is still shorter. Domestic cattle show the first sign of age, a yellow discoloration of the teeth, when five years old. In the sixteenth to eighteenth year the teeth fall out, or break, and the cow ceases to give milk, whilst the bull has lost reproductive power. According to Brehm, cattle live for 25 to 30 years or more. Although the duration of life is short, cattle are not prolific. The gestation period of a cow approaches that of the human race (242–287 days), and there is only one birth a year. The total period of reproductivity lasts only a few years.

The sheep, another domesticated Ruminant, has a life even shorter. According to Grindon, sheep do not live longer than 12 years as a rule, but may reach 14 years, which in their case would be extreme age, as they generally lose their teeth at from 8 to 10 years.

Some Ruminants, such as camels and deer, apparently live longer than sheep or cattle, but I do not know exact facts about them.

The short life of domesticated carnivorous animals is well known. Dogs seldom live more than 16 or 18 years, and even before that, at an age of from 10 to 12, they usually show plain signs of senility. Jonatt has mentioned as an extreme rarity a dog of 22 years of age, and Sir E. Ray Lankester (*Comparative Longevity*, p. 60) cites another instance, in this case the age being 34 years. The oldest dog that I have been able to procure died at the age of 22.

It is generally believed that cats do not live so long as dogs. The average age which they may attain is usually thought to be 10 or 12 years, but certainly a cat of that age has not the decrepid appearance of an old dog. Thanks to the kindness of M. Barrier, the Director of the Ecole d'Alfort, I have had in my possession a cat 23 years old. It appeared to be quite vigorous, and died from cancer in the liver.

Most rodents, particularly the domesticated kinds, are extremely prolific and very short lived. It is extremely rare for a rabbit to reach the age of 10 years, whilst 7 years is the utmost limit for a guinea-pig. Mice, so far as I can ascertain, do not live more than 5 or 6 years.

It is plain from the facts that I have brought together, that mammals, whether they are large or small, as a rule, have shorter lives than birds. It is probable, therefore, that there is something in the structure of mammals which has brought about a shortening in the duration of their lives.

Whilst most of the lower vertebrates, and all birds, reproduce by laying eggs, the vast majority of mammals are viviparous. As the tax on the parent organism is greater when the young are produced alive than when eggs are laid, it might be thought that in this difference lay the cause of the shorter life of mammals. It is well known that an animal may be made feeble by too great fecundity, and it is conceivable that the kind of parasitic life of the embryos within the body of the mother may weaken her system.

There are many facts, however, which make it impossible to accept such a view. The longevity of mammals is nearly equal in the two sexes, although the tax on the organism caused by reproduction is much greater in the case of females than in males. Longevity, however, cannot be regarded as a character stable in each species and necessarily identical in the two sexes. The animal kingdom presents many cases of disparity in this respect, the difference in longevity in the two sexes being specially striking in species of insects. Generally, the females live longer than the males, as, for instance, amongst the Strepsiptera, where the females have 64 times the duration of life of the males. On the other hand, amongst butterflies, there are cases (*e.g.*, *Aglia tau*) where the males live longer than the females. In the human race, there is a difference in the longevity of the sexes, the females having the advantage.

As in most cases of disparity in the duration of life the female lives longer than the male, it is plain that the difference cannot be assigned to the drain on the organism caused by reproduction, which, of course, is much greater in females.

Moreover, a closer scrutiny of the facts shows that although mammals do not live so long as birds, the reproductive drain is greater in the case of birds.

It is well known that the productivity of an animal is not necessarily identical with its fecundity. Fish or frogs which lay thousands of eggs at a time (a pike, for example, produces 130,000) are obviously more prolific than, for instance, a sparrow which lays only 18 eggs in a year, or than a rabbit, which in the same time gives birth to from 25 to 50. However, to produce this much smaller quantity of eggs or of young, the sparrow and the rabbit (I have chosen the most prolific bird and mammal) expend a much larger quantity of material than the frog or the fish. The sparrow and the rabbit employ in producing their progeny a bulk of material greater than the weight of their body, whilst the enormous quantity of eggs laid by the frog does not weigh more than one-seventh part of the body of the frog. It may be laid down, as a general rule, that although fecundity, that is to say the number of eggs or of young which are produced, diminishes as the organism becomes more complex, the productivity on the other hand increases, expressed in percentage of weight. The productivity, which is not more than 18 per cent. in batrachia, reaches 50 per cent. in reptiles, 74 per cent. in mammals, and 82 per cent. in birds.

It is plain that if reproduction shortens the life of mammals by weakening the organism, it must be the productivity, not the fecundity, which is the important factor. I have just shown that productivity is greater in birds than in mammals, and in consequence it cannot be on account of any greater burden of reproduction that mammals have a shorter life than birds. The shortness of mammalian life, again, cannot be attributed to the fact that mammals give birth to young, whilst the long-lived reptiles and birds produce eggs, because the longevity of the males, which produce neither young nor eggs, is none the less practically equal to that of the females of the same species. The reason of the short life of mammals must be sought for elsewhere.

III

THE DIGESTIVE SYSTEM AND SENILITY

Relations between longevity and the structure of the digestive system—The Cæca in birds—The large intestine of mammals—Function of the large intestine—The intestinal microbes and their agency in producing auto-intoxication and auto-infection in the organism—Passage of microbes through the intestinal wall

WE have seen that the duration of life in mammals is relatively shorter than that in birds, and in the so-called "cold-blooded" vertebrates. No indication as to the cause of this difference can be found in the structure of the organs of circulation, respiration, or urinary secretion, or in the nervous or sexual apparatus. The key to the problem is to be found in the organs of digestion.

In reviewing the anatomical structure of the digestive apparatus in the vertebrate series, one soon comes to the striking fact that mammals are the only group in which the large intestine is much developed. In fish, the large intestine is the least important part of the digestive tube, being little wider in calibre than the small intestine. Amongst batrachia, where it is a relatively wide sack, it has begun to assume some importance. In several reptiles it is still larger, and may be provided with a lateral out-growth, which is to be regarded as a cæcum. In birds, the large intestine still remains relatively badly developed; it is short and straight. In most birds, at the point where the large intestine passes into the small intestine, there is a pair of cæca, more or less developed. These cæca are absent in climbing birds, such as the wood-pecker, the oriole, and many others. They are reduced to a pair of tiny out-growths in the eagles, sparrow-hawks, and other diurnal birds of prey, and in pigeons, and perching birds. These organs are larger in the nocturnal birds of prey, in gallinaceous birds, and in ducks, etc.[1]

In the large running birds, such as ostriches, rheas, and tinamous, the cæca are relatively largest. Thus, for instance, in a rhea (*Rhea americana*) which I dissected, the cæca were nearly two-thirds as long as the small intestine. The latter was 1·65 m. in length, whereas one of the cæca was 1·01 m., and the other 0·95 m. The weight of the two cæca with their contents was more than 10 per cent. of the total weight of the bird.

Notwithstanding the exceptions, which are relatively rare, the large intestine is badly developed in the case of birds. On the other hand, it reaches its largest size amongst mammals. In these animals, " only the posterior portion of the latter, or rectum, which passes into the pelvic cavity, corresponds to the large intestine of lower Vertebrates; the remaining, and far larger part, must be looked upon as a neomorph, and is called the colon."[2]

Gegenbaur,[3] another well-known authority on compara-

---

[1] J. Maumus, " Les cæcums des oiseaux," *Annales des sciences naturelles*, 902. See also P. Chalmers Mitchell, " On the Intestinal Tract of Birds," *Trans. Linnæan Soc. of London*, vol. viii. part 7, 1901.

[2] Weidersheim, *Elements of the Comparative Anatomy of Vertebrates*, translated by W. Newton Parker, p. 236, 1886.

[3] *Elements of Comparative Anatomy*, English translation by F. Jeffrey Bell, B.A., London, 1878, p. 562.

DIGESTIVE SYSTEM AND SENILITY

tive anatomy, writes as follows on this subject:—" The hind-gut is longest in the Mammalia, where it forms the large intestine, and is distinguished as such, from the mid-gut, or small intestine. Owing to its greater length, it is arranged in coils, so that the terminal portion only has the straight course taken by the hind-gut of other Vertebrata."

The two series of facts are not to be disputed. On the one hand mammals are shorter lived than birds and lower vertebrates, on the other hand the large intestine is much longer in them than in any other vertebrates. Is there here any link of causality, binding the two characters, or is it a mere coincidence?

To answer the question we must turn to the function of the large intestine in vertebrates. In the lower members of the group (fish, batrachia, reptiles, birds, etc.), the large intestine is not more than a mere reservoir for the waste matter in the food. It takes no share in digestion, as that is the function of the stomach and the small intestine. Only the cæcum can be thought to have some digestive property. In reptiles, the lowest vertebrates in which the cæcum is present, it is so little differentiated from the large intestine itself, that it is difficult to assign to it any specialised function. In very many birds, however, the cæca are well separated from the main digestive tube. The food material passes into them in considerable quantities, and is retained there sufficiently long for some digestive process to take place. M. Maumus has found, in the cæca of birds, secretions which can dissolve albumen and invert sugar cane, but he has been unable to make out that the cæcal juice has any action upon fatty matter. Such digestive power, however, is slight, and when M. Maumus removed the cæca in fowls and ducks, no evil consequences followed. As in many birds the cæca are rudimentary and in others absent, it may be inferred that these organs are useless, and are in process of degeneration in the class. The cæca can be regarded as playing an important part in the organism only in the case of large running birds, where they are very highly developed, but we have not precise information as to their digestive function.

The variations in the structure in the large intestine are greater in mammals than in birds. In some mammals, the large intestine is a simple prolongation of the small intestine, similar in calibre and in structure. In these conditions it may fulfil a definite digestive function. Th. Eimer[1] has determined that in insectivorous bats the large intestine digests insects like the small intestine. Such cases, however, are rare. In most mammals the large intestine is sharply separated from the small intestine by a valve, and opens directly into the cæcum which may be very large. In the horse, the cæcum is an enormous bag, cylindrical and tapering, generally well filled, and holding on an average 35 litres. It is equally large in many other herbivorous animals, such as the tapir, the elephant, and most rodents. In such cases, the food remains for a considerable time in the organ and without doubt undergoes some digestive changes. In many other mammals, particularly carnivorous forms, the cæcum may be quite absent, whilst in some, as for instance, the cat and dog, it is very small; in the latter cases its digestive function must be non-existent or insignificant.[2]

As for the large intestine itself, apart from the special

[1] *Virchow's Archiv*, 1869, vol. xlviii. p. 151.
[2] P. Chalmers Mitchell, "On the Intestinal Tract of Mammals," *Trans. Zool. Soc. of London*, vol. xvii. part 5, 1905.

cases, such as bats, it cannot fulfil any notable digestive function. Th. Eimer was unable to find a proof of any such action in rats and mice, and the very many investigations that have been made in the case of man seem to have established the absence of digestive power in the colon.

Dr. Stragesco,[1] in a recent investigation carried out under the direction of the famous Russian physiologist Pawloff, established that, in normal conditions, digestion and assimilation of food are confined almost exclusively to the small intestine in mammals, and that the large intestine plays only the smallest part. It is only in certain diseases of the digestive tract, in which, on account of increased peristaltic action, the contents of the intestine with the digestive juices are passed quickly from the small intestine to the large intestine, that some digestive work is done in the latter organ.

The large intestine (excluding the cæcum), then, cannot be regarded as an organ of digestion, although absorption of the liquids which have been formed in the small intestine, may take place within its walls. It is known that in the large intestine the contents of the gut give up their water and assume the solid form of fæcal matter. However, whilst the mucous membrane of the large intestine rapidly absorbs water, it has not a similar action on other substances.

The question of the extent to which the large intestine can absorb has been closely investigated, because of its practical importance. It sometimes happens that invalids cannot take food by the mouth, so that their life would be in danger if it were not possible to supply them with food

[1] *Travaux de la Société des médecins russes à Saint-Pétersbourg.* September-October, 1905, p. 18 (in Russian).

otherwise. Attempts have been made to inject nutritive substances through the skin, or, and this is a more usual procedure, by the rectum. By such means the organism can be kept alive for a certain time, but the absorbing power of the large intestine is extremely small. According to Czerny and Lautschenberger[1] the entire colon of the human being can absorb no more than 6 grammes of albumen in 24 hours, an amount which, from the point of view of nutrition, is very small. It was thought that the large intestine might more rapidly absorb albuminous material which had been previously digested and transformed to peptones, but the experiments of Ewald[2] showed that even in that case the absorption was very small. According to more recent experiments of Heile,[3] carried out upon dogs which had cæcal fistulas, and in the case of a man who had an artificial aperture in the colon, the large intestine does not absorb undigested white of egg, and absorbs water, cane sugar, and glucose only very imperfectly. The only substances which are rapidly absorbed through the wall of the colon are the alkaline fluids from fæcal matter. It is possible, however, to nourish invalids by rectal injections of certain nutritious substances, the most important of which is milk.[4]

The large intestine, which has really very slight digestive properties and cannot absorb any considerable bulk of nutriment, is an organ which secretes mucus. The latter serves to moisten the solid fæcal material, so aiding in its expulsion.

We must conclude, therefore, that the large intestine, the organ so highly developed in mammals, is an apparatus

[1] *Virchow's Archiv*, 1874, vol. lix, p. 161.
[2] *Zeitschrift f. klinische. Medicin,* 1887, vol. xii.
[3] *Mittheilungen a. d. Grenzgebieten d. Medicin u. Chirurgie*, 1905, vol. xiv.
[4] Aldor, *Centralblatt f. innere Medicin*, 1898, p. 161.

the general function of which is the preparation and elimination of the waste products of digestion. Why should such an organ be so much more developed in mammals than in the other vertebrates?

In answer to the question, I have formed the theory that the large intestine has been increased in mammals to make it possible for these animals to run long distances without having to stand still for defæcation. The organ, then, would simply have the function of a reservoir of waste matter.

Batrachia and reptiles lead a very idle life, and can move slowly, sometimes because they are protected by poison (toads, salamanders, serpents), sometimes because they have a very hard shell (turtles), sometimes because they are extremely powerful (crocodiles). Mammals, on the other hand, have to move very actively to catch their prey, or to escape from their enemies. Such activity has become possible because of the high development of the limbs, and because the capacity of the large intestine makes possible the accumulation of waste matter for a considerable time.

In order to void the contents of the intestines, mammals have to stand still and assume some particular position. Each act of this kind is a definite risk in the struggle for existence. A carnivorous mammal which, in the process of hunting its prey, had to stop from time to time, would be inferior to one which could pursue its course without pausing. So, also, a herbivorous mammal, escaping from an enemy by flight, would have the better chance of surviving the less it was necessary for it to stand still.

According to such a view, the extreme development of the large intestine would supply a real want in the struggle for existence. M. Yves Delage,[1] the well-known biologist,

[1] *L'année biologique*, 7th year, 1902. Paris, 1903, p. 590.

is unable to accept this hypothesis. He thinks that the rectal enlargement would fulfil the purpose, and adds that everyone has seen herbivorous animals pass their excretions whilst running. The rectum of mammals, however, cannot serve as a reservoir for waste matter, because as soon as such matter reaches the rectum it excites the need of excretion. The waste matter accumulates in the large intestine, from which it passes into the rectum at intervals. When it has reached that region, a sensation is caused which leads to defæcation.

M. Delage is not quite definite when he speaks of mammals voiding their excretions whilst they are in motion. A horse, harnessed to a vehicle, may defæcate whilst it is walking or even running slowly. But these animals cannot defæcate when in rapid motion, and competent observers state that horses never do so whilst racing. In zoological gardens, where animals have room to run about, they stand still before emptying the rectum. M. Ch. Debreuil, who keeps antelopes in a very large park at Melun, has noticed that the excreta are always to be found in masses and not scattered about as if they had been discharged by animals in motion. Antelopes, which are animals that run and leap extremely actively, have to come to a standstill before discharging their small pellets of deer-like excreta.

In the struggle for existence, when a mammal is pursuing its prey or escaping its enemy, there is no question of the leisurely movement of a horse harnessed to an omnibus or cab, but the greatest possible activity is necessary. In such circumstances the possession of an organ within which the excreta could accumulate would be of real importance. My theory of the origin of the mammalian large intestine is intrinsically probable.

Although the capacity of the large intestine may

preserve a mammal in emergencies, it is attended with disadvantages that may shorten the actual duration of life.

The accumulation of waste matter, retained in the large intestine for considerable periods, becomes a nidus for microbes which produce fermentations and putrefaction harmful to the organism. Although our knowledge of the subject is far from complete, it is certain that the intestinal flora contains some microbes which damage health, either by multiplying in the organism, or by poisoning it with their secretions. Most of our knowledge on this matter has come from the study of human patients.

Persons have been known who do not defæcate except at intervals of several days, and who, none the less, do not seem to suffer in health. But the opposite result is more common. The retention of fæcal matter for several days very often brings harmful consequences. Organisms which are in a feeble state from some other cause are specially susceptible to damage of the kind referred to. Infants are frequently seriously ill as the result of constipation. Dr. du Pasquier[1] describes such cases in the following words:—" The infant is leaden in hue, with sunken eyes, dilated pupils, and pinched nostrils. The temperature may reach nearly 104° Fahr.; the pulse is rapid, feeble, and often irregular. Restlessness, insomnia, sometimes convulsions, stiffness of the neck and strabism show that the nervous system is being poisoned by toxins, and even collapse may be reached. The foul and dry tongue, the vomiting and fetid discharges show the disturbance of the digestive tract. Very often an eruption appears, as described by Hutinel, chiefly on the back and buttocks, the front of the thighs and fore-arms." The illness may lead to death but is generally cured by simple purging.

[1] *Gazette des Hôpitaux*, 1904, p. 715.

Women in pregnancy and childbirth frequently suffer much as the result of retention of fæcal matter, and physicians are familiar with the symptoms, which have been described as follows by M. Bouchet[1] :—" After normal parturition, in the course of which the usual antiseptic precautions have been fully pursued, and where delivery has been complete and natural, occasionally the patient is seized with chill and headache. The breath is fetid and the tongue foul. The temperature, taken in the axilla, is nearly 101° Fahr. The abdomen is inflated and painful in the umbilical region. Palpation in the iliac fossæ reveals lumps or consolidations along the colon. Thirst is intense, and there is complete anorexy. On questioning, it is found that there has not been defæcation for several days. The treatment consists of purgatives, enemas, and milk diet. In the next few days the bowels are emptied freely, the abdominal pain ceases, the temperature becomes lower, appetite is restored, and the patient recovers."

Those who suffer from affections of the heart, liver, or kidneys are specially susceptible to the evil results of retained fæcal matter. In such patients an error of diet or constipation may bring about most serious consequences.

Such facts are well known to physicians, and it has been established that complete emptying of the lower bowels leads at once to favourable symptoms. From the other side, it has been shown by experiment that artificial retention of the fæces by ligature of the rectum puts the body in a grave condition.

If we collect our knowledge of all the facts, we cannot doubt but that the cause of the evil is multiplication of

[1] *Accidents dus à la Constipation pendant la Grossesse, l'Accouchement et les Suites des Couches.* Thèse, Paris, 1902, p. 32.

microbes in the contents of the large intestine. When the fæcal matter is free from microbes, as is the case with the meconium of the fœtus or new-born infant, it is not a source of danger to the organism. The waste of cells and the secretions which are added to the undigested food cannot do any harm. Amongst the microbes of the gut, there are some that are inoffensive, but others are known to have pernicious properties.

The ill-health which follows retention of fæcal matter is certainly due to the action of some of the microbes of the gut. There are difficulties, however, in determining the precise mode of action of these microbes. It is generally believed that they form poisonous substances which are absorbed by the walls of the intestine and so pass into the system. The phrase auto-intoxication as applied to infants, women in labour, and patients affected with diseases of the heart, liver, or kidneys, is based on this interpretation of the morbid processes involved. Attempts have been made to isolate and study the poisons in question, but there are many difficulties in the way. To distinguish between the actions of the poisons and of the microbes themselves, the latter have been destroyed by heat or by antiseptics, or been removed by filtration. Such methods, however, may alter the poisons and so are inconclusive. MM. Charron and Le Play[1] have tried to obtain exact results by heating the intestinal microbes to a temperature of about 136° Fahr., a process which probably does not seriously deteriorate the microbial poisons. Such material, injected into the veins of rabbits in large quantities, rapidly produced death, or in smaller quantities, proportionate ill-health.

Kukula[2] has tried to produce this toxic action in animals,

[1] *Comptes rendus de l'Académie des Sciences*, Paris, 1905, 10 July, p. 136. [2] *Archiv. f. klinische Chirurgie*, 1901, vol. lxiii, p. 773.

employing microbial secretions obtained from cases of intestinal obstruction. He succeeded in producing serious symptoms, such as vomiting and curvature of the neck and back, in fact, precisely the sequence of events familiar in cases of obstruction of the bowels or other retentions of fæcal matter.

Some of the products of the intestinal flora are undoubtedly toxic, such as the benzol derivatives (phenol, etc.) ammonium and other salts. Many of these toxins have been insufficiently studied, but it is well known that certain of them can be absorbed by the wall of the gut and act as poisons. A well known case is the toxin of botulism which was isolated and studied by M. van Ermenghem.[1] The poison, the product of a microbe which causes serious intestinal disturbance, is so fatal that a single drop given to a rabbit produces death after symptoms similar to those observed in cases of human beings poisoned by stale food. Butyric acid and the products of albuminous putrefaction are amongst the most pernicious of the microbial poisons produced in the large intestine. It is familiar that digestive disturbance is frequently associated with discharges of sulphuretted hydrogen and putrid excreta, and there is no doubt but that the microbes of putrefaction are the cause of these symptoms.

It has been assumed for long that the retention of fæcal matter tends to putrefactive changes in the intestines, and that the evil consequences of constipation are due to this. Recently, however, bacteriologists have criticised this accepted view, on account of the small number of microbes found in the excreta of constipated persons. Strasburger was the first to establish the fact, and his associate, Schmidt,

[1] Kolle u. Wassermann, *Handb. d. pathogenen Mikro-organismen*, vol. ii, 1903, p. 678.

DIGESTIVE SYSTEM AND SENILITY

showed that putrefaction did not follow when readily putrescible substances were infected with material taken from cases of constipation. However, notwithstanding the exactness of these facts, I cannot accept the inference which has been drawn from them. The excreta discharged naturally in cases of constipation do not give a correct indication of the conditions inside the gut; whilst such matter contains few microbes, the substance removed after injection by an enema is extremely rich in bacteria. Moreover, analysis of the urine, in cases of constipation, shows an excess of the sulpho-conjugate ethers which are known to be products of intestinal putrefaction.

Not only is there auto-intoxication from the microbial poisons absorbed in cases of constipation, but microbes themselves may pass through the walls of the intestine and enter the blood. In the maladies that are the result of constipation some of the symptoms recall those of direct infection, and it is highly probable that, if special investigations were made, microbes of intestinal origin would be found in the blood of the sick children and the pregnant or parturient women whose symptoms I have described above.

The question as to the passage of microbes through the intestinal walls is one of the most controversial of bacteriological problems, and there is little agreement in the numerous publications regarding it. None the less, it is far from impossible to get a general idea of what goes on in an intestinal tract richly charged with microbes.

Although the intestinal wall in an intact state offers a substantial obstacle to the passage of bacteria, it is incontestable that some of these pass through it into the organs and the blood. Numerous experiments performed on different kinds of animals (horses, dogs, rabbits, etc.) show that some of the microbes taken with food traverse the wall of the alimentary canal and come to occupy the adjacent lymphatic glands, the lungs, the spleen and the liver, whilst they are occasionally found in the blood and lymph. Discussion has taken place as to whether the passage takes place when the wall of the gut is absolutely intact or only when it is injured to however small an extent. It would be extremely difficult to settle the question definitely, but it is easy to see that it has little practical bearing. It is known that the wall of the gut is damaged extremely easily, so that the bluntest sound can hardly be passed into the stomach without making a wound through which microbes can pass into the tissues and blood. In the ordinary course of life, the delicate wall of the gut must often undergo slight wounding, and the frequent presence of microbes in the mesenteric ganglia of healthy animals shows clearly what takes place.[1]

It is indubitable, therefore, that the intestinal microbes or their poisons may reach the system generally and bring harm to it. I infer from the facts that the more a digestive tract is charged with microbes, the more it is a source of harm capable of shortening life.

As the large intestine not only is the part of the digestive tube most richly charged with microbes, but is relatively more capacious in mammals than in any other vertebrates, it is a just inference that the duration of life of mammals has been notably shortened as the result of chronic poisoning from an abundant intestinal flora.

[1] Ficker, in the *Archiv. für Hygiene*, vol. lii, p. 179, has recently published the results of an investigation into this.

IV

MICROBES AS THE CAUSE OF SENILITY

Relations between longevity and the intestinal flora—Ruminants—The Horse—Intestinal flora of birds—Intestinal flora of cursorial birds—Duration of life in cursorial birds—Flying mammals—Intestinal flora and longevity of bats—Some exceptions to the rule—Resistance of the lower vertebrates to certain intestinal microbes

In the actual state of our knowledge it is impossible to make a final examination of my hypothesis, as there are many factors about which we are incompletely informed. Nevertheless, it is possible to confront the hypothesis with a large number of accurately established facts.

Although the life of most mammals is relatively short, there are to be found in the group some which live relatively long, as well as others whose life is short. The elephant is an example of the long-lived mammals, whilst ruminants are short-lived forms. In the last chapter, I stated that sheep and cattle became senile at an early age, and did not live long. They are striking exceptions to the rule according to which the duration of life is in direct relation with the size and length of the period of growth. The cow, which is much larger than a woman, and the time of gestation of which is about the same, or a little longer, acquires its teeth at four years old, and becomes senile at an early age; it is quite old at between sixteen and seventeen, an age when a woman is hardly adult; at the age of thirty, practically the extreme limit for bovine animals, a woman is in full vigour.

The precocious old age of ruminants, the constitution of which is well understood, and which are carefully tended, coincides with an extraordinary richness of the intestinal flora. Food remains for a long time in the complicated stomach of these animals, and afterwards the digested masses remain still longer in the large intestine. According to Stohmann and Weiske,[1] in the case of sheep it is a week until the remains of a particular meal have finally left the body of the animal. The excreta of sheep, normally solid, do not betray any special putrefaction in the intestine, but if the body is opened there is abundant evidence of the process. The intestinal contents are richly charged with microbes and give off a strong odour of putrefaction. It is not surprising that under these conditions, the life of sheep should be short.

Another large herbivorous animal, the horse, also dies young, after a premature old age. Although it does not ruminate and possesses a simple stomach, the process of digestion is slow, and enormous masses of nutritive material accumulate in the huge large intestine. Ellenberger and Hofmeister[2] have shown that food remains in the alimentary canal for nearly four days. It remains in the stomach and the small intestine only 24 hours, but about three times as long in the large intestine. This is remarkably different from what happens in the case of birds, in which there is no stagnation during the passage of food through the digestive canal.

[1] Quoted by Frédericq et Nuel, *Eléments de physiologie humaine*, 4th edition, 1899, p. 256.
[2] Quoted by Frédericq et Nuel, *op. cit.*

The structure of birds is adapted for flight, the body being as light as possible, many of the bones and the cavities of the body containing air-sacs. The absence of a bladder and of a true large intestine prevents the accumulation of excreta, these being ejected almost as rapidly as they are formed. The process of ejection, which takes place often in birds, is not so inconvenient as in mammals. The hind limbs are not used in flight, so that they offer no obstacle to evacuation. Thus birds may discharge their droppings while flying.

Such structure and habits make it not surprising that the alimentary canal of many birds contains only a scanty intestinal flora. Parrots, for instance, which are remarkably long-lived birds, harbour very few microbes in the intestine. The small intestine contains almost none, the rectum so few that the fæcal matter appears to be formed of mucus, the waste of the food, and only a very few microbes. M. Michel Cohendy, who has examined the intestinal flora at the Pasteur Institute, was unable to isolate more than five different species of microbes living in the alimentary canal of parrots.

Even in birds of prey which feed upon putrid flesh, the number of microbes in the intestine is remarkably limited. I have investigated the case of ravens which I fed on flesh which was putrid and swarming with microbes. The droppings contained very few bacteria, and it was specially remarkable that the intestines had not the slightest smell of putrefaction. Although the opened body of a herbivorous mammal, such as a rabbit, gives off a strong smell of putrefaction, the body of a raven with the digestive tube exposed has no unpleasant smell. This absence of putrefaction in the intestine is probably the reason of the great longevity of such birds as parrots, ravens, and their allies.

It might be said, however, that the long duration of life in birds is due to the organisation of these animals, rather than to the scantiness of their intestinal flora. To meet this objection, it is necessary to turn to the case of cursorial birds.

There are some birds incapable of flight, the wings of which are badly developed, but which have strong limbs, and can run with great rapidity. Ostriches, cassowaries, rheas, and tinamous, are well known examples of cursorial birds. They live on the surface of the ground, and their habits resemble those of mammals. When they are attacked by enemies, they escape by running so quickly that some of them (ostriches and rheas) outstrip even a horse. However, like mammals, they cannot discharge their secretions when they are running quickly. Tinamous (*Rhynchotus rufescens*), which I have observed in captivity, however quickly they may be running, stop abruptly to discharge their excretions. M. Debreuil, at my request, made observations on this matter, and assured me that the tinamous and rheas (*Rhea americana*) in his park always stood still for this purpose. He has noticed that the droppings, however abundant, were always deposited in heaps. With regard to ostriches, M. Rivière, director of the experimental Gardens at Hamma, Algeria, has been kind enough to give me the following information. " The discharge of excreta," he said in a letter in January, 1901, " is less frequent than in other birds, but the comparatively small size of the enclosures here makes it impossible for me to assert that the animal could discharge its droppings if it were running for a length of time; *a priori* I should think that this did not happen. Normally the bird stands still for defæcation, the tuft of feathers on the tail is lifted up, and there is a violent contraction of the abdominal muscles

MICROBES AS THE CAUSE OF SENILITY

before the sphincters of the cloaca are suddenly opened to discharge the excrement with violence."

I believe that the remarkable development of the large intestine in these running birds has been acquired to obviate the danger which is caused by the animal having to stop for defæcation. Although the huge cæca of these birds have a digestive function, particularly on plants rich in cellulose, I cannot think that the cæca of cursorial birds have been developed for digestion. As a matter of fact, some birds which are not cursorial live on the same kind of food (herbage, seeds, and insects) and have much smaller

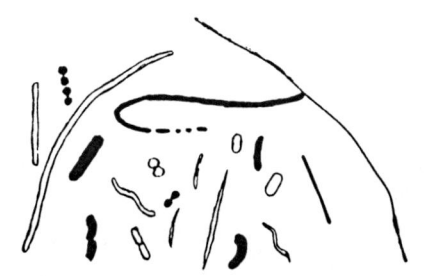

FIG. 14.—Intestinal microbes from the cæca of a Rhea.

cæca, the cæca indeed, in some, for instance, the pigeons, being quite rudimentary.

It is not surprising that the accumulation of food material in the large intestine of running birds is associated with the presence of an extremely rich intestinal flora. Microscopic examination of the excrement of such birds shows this at once. Although the intestinal contents and excrement of many other birds show the presence of very few microbes, belonging to a small number of species, the same materials taken from running birds show enormous quantities of microbes, belonging to a large number of species. In the cæcum of the rhea (Fig. 14) there are bacterial threads, spirilla, bacilli, vibrios, and many kinds of cocci. In the tinamous, the intestinal flora is if possible even richer. According to the statistical investigations of M. Michel Cohendy, the quantity of intestinal microbes in cursorial birds is not less than that found in mammals, even in man.

If I am correct in the view that I have been explaining, cursorial birds, on account of their rich intestinal flora, ought to have a shorter duration of life than that of flying birds. I will now turn to this side of the question. Amongst cursorial forms, there are some of the largest living birds, ostriches being actually the largest living birds, whilst an extinct running bird, the *Aepyornis* of Madagascar, was the largest known bird. According to the rule that large animals live longer than small animals, ostriches should be able to reach a great age. The facts, however, are against this. M. Rivière, who rears ostriches in Algeria, and has a great experience of them, writes to me as follows: " I have no confidence in the stories about the longevity of the ostrich which were told me in the Sahara; they rest on no facts. My personal observation is not very large, but it is quite exact. Some of the ostriches which have been hatched here have lived for 26 years. I do not estimate the duration of life of this bird at more than 35 years, and only one case of this age have I seen myself in 20 years. The bird was a female, a good layer and sitter; she died of old age, showing all the signs of decrepitude, the skin excoriated and lumpy, the feathers degenerate and dry. The bird laid eggs until nearly the end of her life, but at irregular intervals, and the shells were granular instead of being smooth and polished."

In a farm near Nice, where ostriches are reared, there was recently an old male called " Kruger," which was supposed

MICROBES AS THE CAUSE OF SENILITY

to be 50 years old.[1] Countess Stackelberg has been good enough to try to get information for me about this, and informs me that although they have not exact knowledge at the farm, they believe that it must be 50 years old. M. Rivière thinks this statement very surprising, and has nothing in his own long experience to confirm it.

The facts which I have been able to get together do not attribute a long life to other running birds. Gurney mentions that a cassowary (*Casuarius westermanni*) lived 26 years in the Zoological Gardens of Rotterdam, and that three Australian emus (*Dromaeus novae-hollandiae*) had lived in the same Gardens for 28, 22, and 20 years. M. Oustalet (*Ornis*, 1899, vol. x, p. 62) mentions another emu of the same species which died in London at the age of over 23 years. The rhea (*Rhea americana*), another large running bird, does not live so long. "Boecking thinks that its duration of life should be set down at from 14 to 15 years. According to him, many of these birds die of old age" (Brehm, *Oiseaux*, vol. ii, p. 517).

It is striking to compare the short life of cursorial birds, which nevertheless thrive and reproduce in captivity, with the remarkable longevity of so many other birds (parrots, birds of prey) which, although they are much smaller, have been kept alive for from 80 to 100 years. It would be difficult to find a more striking argument in favour of the view that richness of the intestinal flora shortens life. When birds become adapted to terrestrial life and acquire a huge large intestine in which microbes can abound, their duration of life is diminished.

Just as some birds, losing the aerial mode of life, have come to resemble mammals, so also some mammals have

[1] *L'aviculture* (a fortnightly Russian journal), Oct. 1st, 1904, No. 19, p. 3.

become flying animals, provided with wings and in some respects resembling birds. Bats are the most familiar instance. The large intestine, which is extremely useful to running animals, not only ceases to be an advantage but is harmful to flying creatures, insomuch as it increases the weight of the body uselessly. Bats, accordingly, have no cæcum whilst the large intestine is changed in structure and function. Instead of being a capacious tube, serving as a reservoir for the refuse of the food, the large intestine of bats has the same diameter as the small intestine. Its structure is nearly identical. It is provided with glands, and as I have already mentioned in the last chapter, it digests the food in the same way as the small intestine. In fact, the large intestine has become simply a part of the small intestine, the total length of the gut being reduced. Bats, therefore, can no longer retain their secretions but have to empty the intestine almost as often as most birds. I find that Indian fruit bats (*Pteropus medius*) discharge their excreta very often. Microscopic examination shows that there is an absence of microbes quite unusual in the case of a mammal. The alimentary canal of bats is nearly aseptic, containing only a few single bacteria. I have fed these fruit bats with the same food (carrots) which I have given to rabbits, guinea pigs, and mice; whilst the bats accomplished the process of digestion in $1\frac{1}{2}$ hours, and deposited excreta containing fragments of carrot, the rodents took very much longer for digestion and large quantities of waste matter accumulated in the cæca. The intestinal flora too, although the food in each case was the same, showed remarkable differences in these animals. It was almost absent in the bats, whilst in the rabbits, guinea-pigs and mice it consisted of a mass of microbes of different species. The excrement of the bats had no unpleasant odour, and the digestive canal of these bird-like mammals was free

MICROBES AS THE CAUSE OF SENILITY

from putrefaction. Fruit bats fed upon fruit discharged excreta with a pleasant odour of apples and bananas. We have seen that birds which live a life similar to that of mammals acquire a rich intestinal flora and do not live so long as aerial birds. It would be extremely interesting to ascertain the duration of life of bats, mammals which live like birds and have a very scanty intestinal flora. I have been unable to get any exact information as to the duration of life of the true bats, that is to say, the insectivorous bats, as all the requests that I have addressed to specialists have proved fruitless. It appears, however, that it is a popular belief that bats live long. There is a Flemish phrase: " as long-lived as a bat," and a similar phrase is common in Little Russia.

As for the fruit-eating bats, I have been able to ascertain that even in captivity, where the conditions are unfavourable to them, the duration of life is relatively long. I have had in my own possession a fruit bat (*Pteropus medius*) which was bought in Marseilles 14 years ago. It showed no signs of old age, and the teeth were in perfect condition. It died of some acute disease accidentally contracted. I know of another bat of the same species which lived in captivity for more than 15 years, and I have been informed that[1] in the London Zoological Gardens, a fruit bat has lived for 17 years. If these bats were adult when caught, it would be necessary to add something to the known figures.

Although I do not know the exact duration of the life of bats, it is clearly relatively long for mammals no bigger than guinea-pigs. The difference is remarkable if we compare it with the life of sheep, dogs and rabbits, mammals very much larger in size, but possessed of a rich intestinal flora.

The series of facts that I have been discussing strengthens

[1] *Country Life*, 1905.

my conviction that the intestinal flora is an extremely important factor in the causation of senility. It must not be supposed, however, that all the known facts can be explained equally easily on this hypothesis. The harm done by microbes cannot always be measured by their abundance in the alimentary canal. In the first place, it must be remembered that some microbes are useful; moreover, microbes, even although their products are very dangerous, may exist in quantities in an organism, and yet do no harm if the organism has the power of resisting bacterial poisons. Thus, for instance, the bacillus of tetanus, which thrives in the alimentary canal, and which can endanger life if the wall of the gut is wounded, does not harm a crocodile or a tortoise, as these animals are extremely resistant to the poison of tetanus. Dr. Favorsky, by experiments at the Pasteur Institute, has shown that the poison of botulism can be absorbed with impunity by some birds, and by tortoises, although death follows if a very small quantity of it be introduced into the alimentary canal of a mammal.

The bodies of man and of higher animals are possessed of a complex mechanism which resists the harmful action of bacteria and their poisons. The various parts of this mechanism may act differently, with the result that there is great variation in the power of resistance. Thus, however abundant microbes may be in the intestine, they may bring little harm to an organism that has a high power of destruction or neutralisation of the toxins, or when these harmful products are unable to pass through the intestinal wall. It is in this way that I explain some exceptions to the general rule, which are exceptions only in appearance. Such a case is that of the nocturnal birds of prey. Although the diurnal birds of prey (eagles, vultures, etc.) have very short cæca, in which the food is never found, owls have very large

MICROBES AS THE CAUSE OF SENILITY

cæca, which may be as long as 10 cm. (Eagle-Owl, *Bubo maximus*). These long cæca, however, contain debris of the food only in the enlarged terminal portion, and the food masses contain a very small number of microbes. Notwithstanding a great difference in the length of the cæca between the owls and the eagles, these two groups of birds do not differ greatly in longevity. But the difference in the cæca does not imply a corresponding difference in the intestinal flora which appears to be very scanty in both cases.

It is possible that the elephant is a more real exception to the rule. Here is a case of a mammal with an enormous large intestine and a capacious cæcum, and which none the less is capable of surviving for a century. I have had no opportunity of investigating the elephant from this point of view, and have no explanation to suggest.

Monkeys and man differ from most mammals in so far as they possess a long duration of life, although their large intestines are very capacious. I have been unable to get exact information as to the longevity of monkeys, but I understand that these animals live longer than domesticated mammals, such as the ox, sheep, dog, and cat. Anthropoid apes are supposed to be able to reach the age of 50 years. The only other mammal with a longevity similar to that of the elephant is man.

V

DURATION OF HUMAN LIFE

Longevity of man—Theory of Ebstein on the normal duration of human life—Instances of human longevity—Circumstances which may explain the long duration of human life

MAN has inherited from his mammalian ancestors his organisation and qualities. His life is notably shorter than that of many reptiles, but longer than that of many birds and most other mammals. None the less he has inherited a capacious large intestine in which a most abundant intestinal flora flourishes.

Gestation and the period of growth are long in the human race, and from the point of view of theoretical considerations, human longevity should be longer than it generally is. Haller, a distinguished Swiss physiologist of the 18th century, thought that man ought to live to 200 years; Buffon was of the opinion that when a man did not die from some accident or disease he would reach 90 or 100 years.

According to Flourens, man takes 20 years to grow and ought to live 5 times 20, that is to say, 100 years.

The actual longevity is much below these figures, which are based on theory. I have shown, moreover, that even if the rule based on the theory of growth can be accepted as generally true, it cannot be applied in every case, as the factors controlling duration of life are very variable.

Statistics show that the highest human mortality occurs in the earliest years of life. In the first year after birth alone, one quarter of the children die. After this period of maximum mortality, the death-rate slowly falls until the age of puberty, and then rises again slowly and continuously. It reaches a second maximum between the ages of 60 and 75, and then slowly falls again to the extreme limit of longevity.

Bodio,[1] an Italian man of science, holds the view that the great mortality of infants is a natural adaptation to prevent too great an increase of the human race. This view, however, cannot be supported, and rational hygiene readily brings about a great diminution in the mortality of children. The cause of mortality is in most cases maladies of the intestinal canal, produced by erroneous diet, and with the advance of civilisation, infant mortality has been very greatly reduced.

I find it impossible to accept the view that the high mortality between the ages of 70 and 75 indicates a natural limit of human life. As a result of investigations into mortality in most of the European countries, Lexis came to the conclusion that the normal duration of human life was not more than 75 years. Dr. Ebstein[2] accepts this statistical result and announces that " we now know the normal limit set by nature to the life of mankind. This limit is at the age of maximum mortality. If man dies before then, his death is premature. Everyone does not reach the normal limit; life ends generally before it, and only in rare cases after it."

The fact that many men of from 70 to 75 years old are well preserved, both physically and intellectually, makes

[1] Quoted by Ebstein, *Die Kunst d. mensch. Leben zu verlängern*, 1891.
[2] *Op. cit.*, p. 12.

it impossible to regard that age as the natural limit of human life. Philosophers such as Plato, poets such as Goethe and Victor Hugo, artists such as Michael Angelo, Titian and Franz Hals, produced some of their most important works when they had passed what Lexis and Ebstein regard as the limit of life. Moreover, deaths of people at that age are rarely due to senile debility. In Paris, for instance, in 1902, of cases of deaths between the ages of 70 and 74, only 8·5 per cent. were due to old age.[1] Infectious diseases, such as pneumonia, tuberculosis, diseases of the heart and the kidneys, and cerebral hæmorrhage, caused most of the deaths of these old people. Such cases of death, however, can often be avoided and must be regarded as accidental rather than natural.

Confirmation of the view that the natural limit is not at 70 to 75 years is to be found in the fact that so many men reach a greater age. Centenarians are really not rare. In France, for instance, nearly one hundred and fifty people die every year, after having reached the age of 100 or more. In 1836, in a population of thirty-three millions and a half (33,540,910), there were 146 centenarians, that is to say, one in about 220,000 inhabitants. In some other countries, particularly in Eastern Europe, the number of centenarians is still greater. In Greece, for instance, there is a centenarian for each set of 25,641 living persons, that is to say, nine times as many as in France.[2]

What age can be reached by the human species? Formerly it was supposed that individuals might live for several centuries; to say nothing of Methuselah, whose age of 969 years, mentioned in the Bible, is the result of a mistake in calculation, I may mention Nestor, who, accord-

[1] *Annuaire statistique de la ville de Paris*, 23rd year, 1904, p. 164-171.
[2] Ornstein, Virchow's *Archiv.*, 1891, vol. cxxv, p. 408.

ing to Homer, lived for three human ages, that is to say, 300 years, or Dando, the Illyrian, and the King of the Lacmons, who were supposed to have reached ages of five or six centuries. These ancient records are, of course, quite incorrect. Much more confidence can be placed in some facts relating to more modern times, according to which the extreme old age reached by man was 185 years. Kentigern, the founder of the Cathedral of Glasgow, known by the name of St. Mungo, died at the age of 185, on Jan. 5th, 600.[1] Another astonishing case of longevity is related from Hungary, where an agriculturist, Pierre Zortay, born in 1539, died in 1724. The Hungarian records of the 18th century contain other cases of death at ages between 147 and 172 years.

The case of Drakenberg is still more authentic; he was born in Norway in 1626 and died in 1772, at the age of 146. He was known as the Old Man of the North. He had been captured by African pirates and was held by them for fifteen years, and was engaged as a sailor for ninety-one years. His romantic history attracted contemporary attention; and the journals of the time (*Gazette de France*, 1764, *Gazette d'Utrecht*, 1767, etc.)[2] contain information regarding him. The well-known instance of Thomas Parr appears to rest on good authority. Parr was a poor Shropshire peasant, who did hard work until he was 130 years old, and who died in London at the age of 152 years and 9 months. The celebrated Harvey examined the body after death and was unable to discover organic disease; even the cartilages of the ribs were not ossified and were elastic as in a young man. The brain, however, was hard and resisting to the touch, as its blood-vessels were

[1] Ebstein, *op. cit.*, p. 70.
[2] Lejoncourt, *Galerie des centenaires*, Paris, 1842, p. 96-98.

thickened and dry. Parr was buried in Westminster Abbey.[1]

It appears, then, that human beings may reach the age of 150, but such cases are certainly extremely rare, and are not known from the records of the last two centuries. I cannot accept without a good deal of reserve the statements as to two persons who died in the beginning of the 19th century at the ages of 142 and 145. On the other hand, cases of duration of life from 100 to 120 years are not very rare.

Extreme longevity is not limited to the white races. According to Prichard,[2] negroes have lived respectively to 115, 160, and 180 years. In the course of the 19th century there have been observed, in Senegal, eight negroes ranging from 100 to 121 years old. M. Chemin[3] saw himself in 1898 at Foundiougne an old man, whom the natives stated to be 108 years of age; although he was in good health, he had been blind for several years. The same author, on the authority of the *New York Herald* of June 13th, 1895, mentions the case of a coloured woman in North Carolina, who was more than 140 years old, and of a man 125 years old.

Women more frequently become centenarians than men, although the difference is not very great. For instance, in Greece, in 1885, in a population of nearly two millions (1,947,760), there were 278 persons aged from 95 to 110 years, of whom 133 were male and 145 female.

[1] Lejoncourt, *op. cit.*, p. 101.
[2] *Researches into the Physical History of Mankind*, 1836, vol. i, p. 1157.
[3] I owe to the kindness of M. Chemin a memoir in which he has brought together the ancient and new records on the centenarians of all countries up to the end of the nineteenth century. M. Chemin was unable to find a publisher, but has given me his manuscript, extending to 182 pages.

In the seven years, from 1833 to 1839 inclusive, according to Chemin, there were in Paris twenty-six men over the age of 95, and forty-five women. Such facts, and many others, support the general proposition that male mortality is always greater than that of the other sex.

In most cases centenarians are notably healthy and of strong constitution. There are instances, however, of abnormal people having reached a great age. A woman, called Nicoline Marc, died in 1760, at the age of 110. Since she was two years old, her left arm was crippled. Her hand was bent under the arm like a hook. She was a hunch-back, and so bent that she appeared to be no more than four feet high. A Scotch woman, Elspeth Wilson, died at the age of 115 years. She was quite a dwarf, being only a little over two feet high. On the other hand, although they usually have a very short life, giants have been known to reach the age of 100.

Haller, in the eighteenth century, remarked that centenarians often occurred in the same family, as if longevity were a hereditary quality. It is certainly the case that the descendants of centenarians frequently reach extreme age. Thomas Parr, for instance, left a son who died in 1761, at the age of 127 years, having retained his mental faculties until death. In M. Chemin's list of centenarians, there are eighteen cases of extreme old age having been reached by their relations. As all innate characters can be transmitted, the influence of heredity and longevity must be admitted. At the same time, it is necessary to remember the important influence of the similarity of conditions in the case of parents and children. Many cases of tuberculosis and leprosy, which used to be assigned to heredity, are now known to be due to infection in the same conditions of life, and some of the examples of the attaining of a great age by more than one member of a family may be explained by the influence of surrounding circumstances. Very frequently the husband and wife, although not related by blood, both attain extremely advanced age. I found 22 cases of this kind in M. Chemin's list; I will give a few of them. A widow, Anne Barak, died at the age of 123, in Moravia; her husband died at the age of 118. In 1896, there was alive in Constantinople, M. Christaki, a retired army doctor of the age of 110; his wife was 95 years old. In 1886, M. et Mme. Gallot, aged respectively 105 years and 4 months, and 105 years and one month, died within two days of each other at Vaugirard, 54, Rue Cambronne. Lejoncourt mentions a South American of 143 years old, whose wife had lived to the age of 117.

It is worth enquiring if there be any relation between longevity and locality. There are some countries in which very many of the natives reach old age. It appears that Eastern Europe (Balkan States, and Russia), although its civilisation is not high, contains many more centenarians than Western Europe. I have already mentioned that Dr. Ornstein had shown the existence of many extremely old people in Greece. M. Chemin states that in Servia, Bulgaria and Roumania there were more than 5,000 centenarians (5,545) living in 1896. "Although these figures appear to be exaggerated," wrote M. Chemin, "it is undoubtedly the case that the pure and keen air of the Balkans, and the pastoral or agricultural life of the natives, predisposes to old age." The same author mentions several localities in France, notable for the numbers of very old people. In 1898 in the commune of Sournia (Pyrénées-Orientales) the total population was 600, amongst which there was one woman of 95 years, a man of 94, a woman of 89, two men of 85, two of 84, and two of

83, three women of 82, and two men of 80. At St. Blimont in the Department of the Somme, amongst the 400 inhabitants alive in 1897, there were six men between the ages of 85 and 93 years and one woman in her 101st year.

It cannot be accepted that it is the keen air which lengthens the life, because Switzerland, a mountainous country, is notable for the rarity of centenarians. It is more likely that some circumstance in the mode of living influences longevity.

It has been noticed that most centenarians have been people who were poor, or in humble circumstances, and whose life has been extremely simple. There are instances of rich centenarians, such as Sir Moses Montefiore who died at the age of 101, but such are extremely rare. It may well be said that great riches do not bring a very long life. Poverty generally brings with it sobriety, especially in old age, and it has been often said that most centenarians have lived an extremely sober life. They have not all followed the example of the celebrated Cornaro, who brought himself to subsist on a daily diet of no more than twelve ounces of solid food, and fourteen ounces of wine, and who, although his constitution was weak, lived for about a century. He has left extremely interesting Memoirs, and retained his intelligence until his death on the 26th April, 1566 (Lejoncourt, p. 146).

In M. Chemin's list I have counted twenty-six centenarians, distinguished by their frugal life. Most of them did not drink wine, and many of them limited themselves to bread, milk and vegetables.

Sobriety is certainly favourable to long life, but it is not necessary, because quite a number of centenarians have drunk freely. Several of those who are catalogued by Chemin, drank wine and spirits even to excess. Catherine Reymond, for instance, who died in 1758 at the age of 107 years, drank much wine, and Politiman, a surgeon who lived from 1685 to 1825, was in the habit, from his twenty-fifth year onwards, of getting drunk every night, after having attended to his practice all day. Gascogne, a butcher of Trie (Hautes-Pyrénées), died in 1767 at the age of 120, and had been accustomed to get drunk twice a week. A most curious example is that of the Irish land-owner Brawn, who lived to the age of 120, and who had an inscription put upon his tombstone that he was always drunk, and when in that condition was so terrible that even death had been afraid of him. Some districts, even, are distinguished at once for the longevity of their inhabitants and for the large local consumption of alcohol. In 1897, the village of Chailly in the Côte-d'Or had no less than twenty octogenarians amongst 523 inhabitants. This village is one of the localities in France where most alcohol is consumed, and the old people are very far from being distinguished from their younger fellows by any special sobriety.

In some cases centenarians have been much addicted to the drinking of coffee. The reader will recall Voltaire's reply when his doctor described the grave harm that comes from abuse of coffee which acts as a real poison. " Well," said Voltaire, " I have been poisoning myself for nearly 80 years." There are centenarians who have lived longer than Voltaire, and have drunk still more coffee. Elisabeth Durieux, a native of Savoy, reached the age of 114. Her principal food was coffee, of which she took daily as many as forty small cups. She was jovial and a boon table companion, and used black coffee in quantities that would have surprised an Arab. Her coffee-pot was always on the fire, like the tea-pot in an English cottage (Lejoncourt, p. 84; Chemin, p. 147).

It has been noticed that many centenarians do not smoke,

but this like all other traits is not universal. M. Ross, who gained a prize for longevity in 1896 at the age of 102, was an inveterate smoker. In 1897, a widow named Lazennec, died at La Carrière, in Kérinou, Finistère, at the age of 104. She lived in a hovel on charity, and she had smoked a pipe ever since she was quite young.

It is plain that any factor to which long duration of life has been attributed disappears when many cases are examined. Naturally a sound constitution and a simple and sober life are favourable to longevity, but apart from these, there is something unknown which tends to long life. The celebrated physiologist of Bonn, Pflüger,[1] came to the conclusion that the chief condition of longevity is something "intrinsic in the constitution," something which cannot be defined exactly, and which must be set down to inheritance.

In the present state of knowledge, we cannot denote the chief cause of human longevity, but the proper course will be to seek it out as we would seek out that of animal longevity. As human longevity is often local in its character, and is exhibited by married people who have nothing in common except their mode of life, we may enquire into the intestinal flora and the mechanism by which the organism resists its harmful effect as factors which influence the duration of life. It is reasonable to suppose that in persons living in the same district or under the same roof, the intestinal flora may be similar. The problem can be settled only by a series of laborious researches which have yet to be made. At present I can do no more than bring together a large number of facts regarding the duration of life in man and in animals, with the hope of suggesting the lines for future investigation.

[1] *Ueber die Kunst d. Verlängerung d. mensch. Lebens*, Bonn, 1890, p. 23.

PART III

INVESTIGATIONS ON NATURAL DEATH

I

NATURAL DEATH AMONG PLANTS

Theory of the immortality of unicellular organisms—Examples of very old trees—Examples of short-lived plants—Prolongation of the life of some plants—Theory of the natural death of plants by exhaustion—Death of plants from auto-intoxication

It must surprise my readers to find how little science really knows about death. Although death has a preponderating place in religions, systems of philosophy, literature and folk-lore, scientific works pay little attention to it. This unfortunate fact explains, although it may not justify, the bitter attack made on science on the grounds that it is occupied with minutiæ and neglects the great problems of human life, such as death. When Tolstoi was absorbed by the problem and searched for some solution in the writings of scientific men, he found that the explanations were trivial or inexact. In consequence he was extremely indignant with the men who devoted themselves to the investigation of what seemed to him useless problems (such as the insect world, or the structure of cells and tissues) and who were yet unable to say what the destiny of man or death might be.

I am far from claiming to solve these problems; I can do little more than describe the actual state of the question of natural death. I hope in this way at least to prepare for scientific investigation, and to call attention to it as the most important problem of humanity.

By the use of the phrase "natural death" I mean to denote a phenomenon that is intrinsic in the nature of an organism and that is not the mere result of an external accident. Popular phraseology includes under natural death all cases due to diseases. But as such deaths can be avoided and are not due to qualities inherent in the organism, it is erroneous to include them in the category "natural death."

In nature, death comes so frequently by accident that there is justification for asking if natural death really occurs. It used to be thought that death was the inevitable end of life and that the living principle contained within itself the germ of death. Accordingly, it was a surprising discovery that many low organisms die only by accident, and that if such accident be avoided, death does not fall on them. Unicellular organsims (such as infusoria, many other protozoa and low plants) multiply by simple division, the organism thus giving rise to two new organisms; the parent so to speak loses itself in its offspring without undergoing death. To criticisms of this mode of presentment of the facts, Weismann, who has attracted most attention to the view, replied as follows:—"In cultures of Infusoria, these little animals continually multiply by division and no dead bodies are found. The individual life is short, but it ends not in death but in transformation to two new individuals."

Max Verworn,[1] a physiologist of repute, objected that Weismann had overlooked the occurrence within the organism of a process of partial destruction, and that under certain conditions a complete organ of the infusorian body (the nucleus) dies and is absorbed. Such death of a part, however, is not followed by death of the whole, and as the

[1] *Physiologie générale*, 1900, p. 381.

continuous destruction of some of the cells in our own bodies is not regarded as our death, the criticism of the German physiologist cannot be accepted.

It is not only the extremely short-lived microscopic organisms that escape death. Some of the higher plants, which may attain to gigantic size, encounter death only by accidents. There is nothing to be found in the nature of their organisation which would seem to indicate that death is the inevitable or even probable result of their constitutions.

The longevity of some trees has long been notorious, as these appear to live for many centuries and to die only when they are overwhelmed by the ravages of a storm or killed by human agency.

When the Canary Islands were discovered, in the beginning of the fifteenth century, the early explorers were struck with the gigantic size of a dragon tree which was venerated by the natives as their tutelary deity. The tree stood in a Garden at Orotava in Teneriffe, and even in these early days, its huge trunk contained a gigantic hollow. The tree did not reward the worship of the natives, who were annihilated by the Spaniards, and it survived them for nearly four centuries. At the end of the eighteenth century it was seen by Humboldt,[1] who found that the trunk was forty-five feet in circumference, and who attributed to it a great age because dragon trees grow extremely slowly. Early in the nineteenth century (1819) a furious tempest swept over Orotava and with a gigantic crash nearly a third of the crown of leaves and branches fell on the ground. Notwithstanding this shock, the monster survived for fifty years. Berthelot,[2] who visited it in 1839, described it as follows:—
" A dragon tree stood in front of my dwelling, grotesque in

[1] *Tableaux de la nature* (French translation), 1808, vol. ii, p. 109.
[2] Webb and Berthelot, *Histoire naturelle des îles Canaries*, 1839, vol. i, part 2, pp. 97-98.

NATURAL DEATH AMONG PLANTS

form, gigantic in size, which a storm had smitten without overwhelming. Ten men would have much ado to girdle

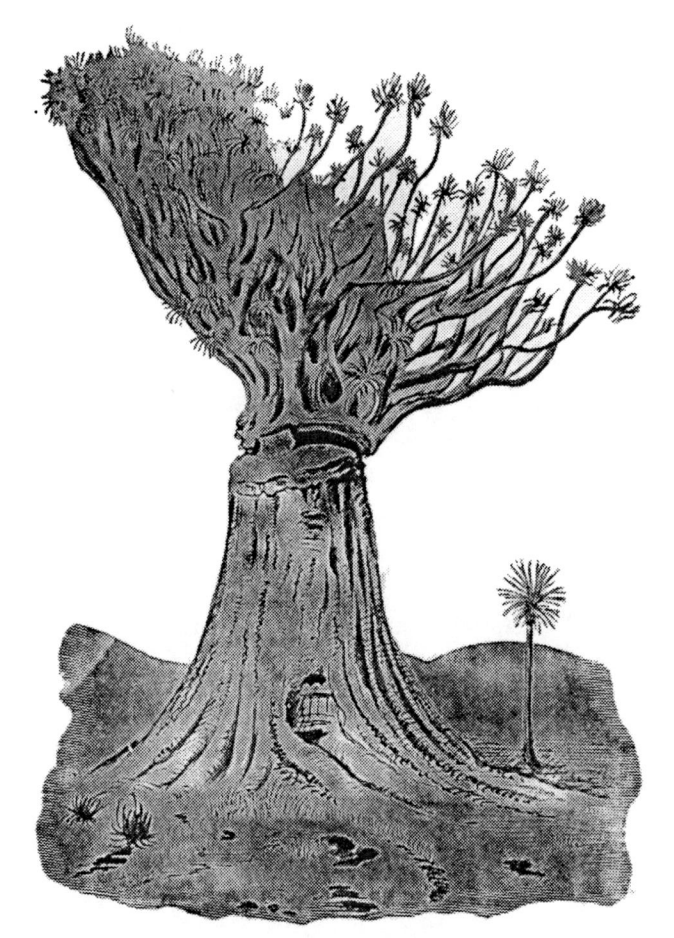

Fig. 15.—The Dragon-tree of the villa Orotava.

its vast trunk, fifty feet in circumference at the ground. The huge column had a deep cave within it, hollowed by the ages; a rustic porch gave access to the interior, and the lofty dome, although half had been destroyed by a storm, still bore an enormous crown of branches."

The famous dragon-tree got more and more damaged, and was finally overthrown by a storm in 1868. A few years after the catastrophe (in 1871) I myself saw the remains of the colossus, lying on the ground as a huge grey mass like some antediluvian monster. No accurate estimate of its age can be formed, but it must have lived several thousand years.

Trees have been known which were still older than the dragon-tree of Teneriffe. One of the best known is the baobab of Cape Verd, described by Adanson. " This remarkable tree was thirty feet in diameter when the famous French naturalist measured and described it. Three centuries earlier, some English sailors had cut an inscription on it, and Adanson laid this bare by removing three hundred layers of wood. On his observations Adanson based an estimate of 5,150 years as the age of the tree.[1] The old cypresses of Mexico are thought to be still older. A. de Candolle[2] concluded that the cypress of Montezuma was 2,000 years old when he saw it, and that the cypress at Oazaca was much older than the tree described by Adanson. In California, trees of the species *Sequoia gigantea* are three thousand years old, and Sargent, an American botanist, attributes to some of them an age of at least five thousand years.

The question of the nature of individuality in the vegetable world has been raised in connection with the longevity of trees. It has been asked if a tree is to be regarded as a single individual or as a colony of many plants like a branching polyp. It is a difficult question, but only of

[1] *Bibliothèque universelle de Genève*, 1839, vol. xlvi. p. 387.
[2] *Ibid.*, p. 392.

secondary importance from the point of view of this discussion. A. de Candolle,[1] having paid special attention to the subject, came to the conclusion that trees do not die of old age, that, in the real sense of the phrase, there is no natural end of their existence. Many botanists agree with him. Naegeli[2] holds that a tree several thousand years old dies only from external accidents.

It is plain that amongst the lower plants and the higher plants there are cases where natural death does not exist. Theoretically, life would have an unlimited duration, subject to the continuous replacement of the substance of the organism in the normal metabolism. It must not be inferred, however, that there is no such occurrence as natural death amongst plants. There are numerous cases where death comes quite apart from the agency of external forces. Even amongst closely related plants there are some cases where natural death does not occur, and others where it is normal. The lower fungi offer a good instance. Some of these pass through a longer or shorter vegetative stage and then the living mass breaks up into spores (*Myxomycetes*). The whole bulk of matter is not transformed, but the remnant consists only of cuticular secretions, not living cells. In other fungi, only some of the cells transform to spores, the others dying naturally.

One stage of the life history of some lower plants is of short duration. The prothalli of some cryptogams (*Marsiliaceæ*) live only a few hours, just long enough for the appearance of the sexual organs. When these are ripe the body of the prothallus and all its constituent cells fall a prey to natural death. In such cases there is a " corpse,"

[1] *Bibliothèque universelle de Genève*, vol. xlvii, p. 49.
[2] *Entstehung u. Begriff d. naturhistorischen Art*, 2nd edit., Munich, 1865, p. 37.

composed of dead cells and protoplasm. Even amongst the higher plants there are instances of an extremely short duration of life. *Amaryllis lutea* passes through all the stages of its life-history in ten days, the minimum time necessary for the sprouting of the leaves and flowers and the production of the seeds, after which it dies naturally.[1] It is interesting to find that in the same family there are other plants notable for long duration of life. The Agave requires a century to produce its flowers before death comes naturally.

Everyone is familiar with the so-called " annual " plants which live only a few months, from the time when they sprout, until, after the production of seed, death comes to them naturally. The life of annuals, however, can be preserved for two or for several years. Rye is normally an annual, but some varieties are able to live for two years and produce two crops. The Cossacks of the Don have established this fact, and have cultivated a biennial variety of rye for many years.[2] Beetroot[3] is normally biennial, but has been changed to a plant which lives for from three to five years. Such instances are by no means unique.

Natural death can be postponed if the plant be prevented from seeding. Professor Hugo de Vries has prolonged the life of the Oenotheras he cultivates, by cutting the flowers before fertilisation. Under ordinary conditions the stem dies after producing from forty to fifty flowers, but, if cutting be practised, new flowers are produced until the winter cold intervenes. By cutting the stem sufficiently early, the plants are induced to develop new buds at the base, and these buds survive winter, and resume growth in the fol-

---

[1] Griesebach, *Die Vegetation der Erde*.

[2] Batalin, *Acta Horti Petropolitani*, vol. xi, no. 6, 1890, p. 289.

[3] I am indebted to Prof. Hugo de Vries for this and other instances of the prolongation of life in plants.

NATURAL DEATH AMONG PLANTS

lowing spring." (Extract from a letter of Prof. H. de Vries.)

The grass of lawns is usually mowed before it begins to flower, so as to prevent the ripening of the seeds and the death of the plant. When this is done, the grass remains continually green, and its life lasts for several years.

The connection between the seeding of plants and their natural death has been recognised for long, and is usually explained as being due to the exhaustion of the plant.

As I am not a botanist, and was anxious to know the views of botanists on natural death, I wrote to Prof. de Vries, as a universally accepted authority. The distinguished botanist replied to me as follows. " Your question is extremely difficult. I do not think that much is known as to the exact cause of the death of annual plants, but it is customary to attribute it to exhaustion." All the botanists who have expressed opinions on this matter appear to hold a similar view. Hildebrand,[1] the author of a memoir on the duration of life in plants, stated this view again and again. According to him " the life of annuals is usually short because they are exhausted by their extensive production of seeds (p. 116)." "Even amongst plants which produce seeds for several years, there are some which are prematurely exhausted by fructification and which die spontaneously " (p. 67). In the prothallus of many of the higher cryptogams, the formation of a single embryo is followed by natural death; as Goebel[2] points out, the embryo completely absorbs the prothallus.

As plants generally obtain their food with ease, it is natural to ask what is the cause of the exhaustion after seeding. When a plant which cannot resist cold dies after it has produced its seeds in the end of the summer, the event

[1] Engler's *Botanische Jahrbücher*, Leipzig, 1882, vol. ii, p. 51.
[2] *Organographie der Pflanzen*, Iéna, 1898-1901.

is natural enough. But how can we explain the death of an annual plant which is growing in a rich soil, and which seeds in the beginning of the summer, as being due to exhaustion long before the winter cold. It frequently happens that after harvest new shoots spring up from grains which have fallen. The soil which can support this new vegetation cannot have been exhausted by the cereal in question; and there has been enough warmth for the new crop. It cannot be the external conditions which have caused the death of the parent plant. The explanation of this apparent contradiction has been sought in the constitution of the plant itself. Hildebrand remarks that "certain species have a constitution which tends to early fructification. As soon as the seeds have been set, the strength of the plant is exhausted in the swelling of the grains, so that the plant dies." "Other species, on the contrary, are so constituted that they vegetate for a long time, before fruiting, after which, however, they also die. A third set of plants have such a constitution that "they do not die after seeding, that they can seed often and live for many years" (p. 113).

Being unable to indicate exactly the intrinsic mechanism of these different "constitutions," several botanists explain them by a kind of teleological predestination. According to Hildebrand "the nutritive processes of a plant have no other purpose than to make it capable of reproduction; this final end, however, can be reached in different modes and after different periods of time" (p. 132). Goebel sets down similar views. "In heterosporous plants the whole course of the development of prothalli is predetermined. The prothalli, so far as we actually know, to use the phrase of theologians, are predestined; their fate is determined once for all" (p. 403). M. Massart[1] expresses the same kind of view, when he says that "some-

[1] *Bulletin du jardin botanique de Bruxelles*, vol. i, no. 6, 1905.

times cells die because their work is finished, and they have no longer any reason for existing."

Such an interpretation of the facts is quite opposed to determinism, and makes the problem of natural death in the plant world more difficult but more interesting.

The modern scientific conception of the universe excludes the idea of predestination. The relations between fructification and natural death must be regulated by the law of selection, according to which no organism survives if its reproduction is impossible. It occasionally happens that children are born without organs which are indispensable to life. Such monsters of different kinds being non-viable, cannot be said to be predestined to death, as they die because of defects in their structure. Others are born with all that is necessary for life, and survive for that reason, not because they are predestined to life. So also species of plants which develop incompletely and which die before they have produced spores or seeds, cannot survive; whilst those which die after having given birth to the next generation survive in their descendants. However quickly death follow the production of seed, the species will survive equally well. The cause of the natural death of plants must be sought, therefore, not in predestination, but in the mechanism of the organic processes.

Nothing seems more probable than that a plant should die when all its organic forces have been exhausted. It would be interesting, however, to ascertain the mechanism of that exhaustion, and this especially because it is often very difficult to imagine a cause for it. Many plants exist which produce several generations each season, in the same soil, without exhausting it. In perennial plants, some parts, such as the flowers, die periodically, although the plant itself is not exhausted. Everyone has seen that in geraniums some of the flowers wither whilst others are blooming, the process going on throughout the season. We can scarcely attribute such a natural death of the flowers to any exhaustion of the plant which continues to produce new flowers.

The fairly frequent prolongation of the life of plants is also out of harmony with the theory of natural death as the result of exhaustion. It sometimes happens that male plants produce female flowers abnormally; cases of this kind have been observed in willows, stinging-nettles, hops, and especially in maize.[1] Here we have to deal with a kind of monstrosity, differing, however, from the non-viable monsters of the human race, in the respect that the production of female flowers on the male branches results in the prolongation of their lives. Generally the male branches die a natural death as soon as the pollen has been shed, and therefore some time before the death of the female flowers. If, however, a male branch bears a female flower which becomes fertilised, then the life of the branch is prolonged until the seeds ripen. If the natural death of the male flowers is the result of exhaustion due to the development of the pollen, how can we reconcile this with the prolongation of life in a case where the male branch has also female flowers to nourish and seeds to mature?

It is quite clear that natural death, in such cases, is the result of a mechanism more complex than simple exhaustion.

Prof. de Vries has already noted that the duration of life in plants depends on their vital processes. That view implies that there are some qualities inherent in its organisation which can prolong or shorten the life of a plant, and it

[1] Hugo de Vries, *Jahrbücher für wissensch. Botanik*, 1890, vol. xxii, p. 52.

is here that we ought to find the key to the problem of natural death in the vegetable world. However, to gain exact knowledge of such factors, it would be necessary to have information on many points in plant physiology which unfortunately are very imperfectly known. In this respect, the vital conditions of the simplest plants, such as yeasts and bacteria, have been investigated much more fully. It is true that such low organisms reproduce freely either by division or by budding, so that they are amongst the organisms in which natural death is not inevitable. None the less, in their lives phenomena occasionally present themselves which can be interpreted as cases of natural death.

At a time when it was still unknown that all fermentation was due to the action of microscopic plants, it had been observed that, in certain conditions, fermentation ceased much more quickly than in other conditions. For instance, when sugar is being transformed to lactic acid, it is useful to add chalk, as otherwise the fermentation stops before the greater part of the sugar has been acted upon. When, in 1857, Pasteur made his great discovery of the lactic acid microbe, he showed that that little organism, although it could produce lactic acid, was interfered with by an excess of the acid. To secure complete fermentation, it was necessary to neutralise the acid by the addition of chalk.

When the action of lactic acid is continued too long, it not only arrests the process of fermentation but definitely kills the microbe. It is for that reason that it has been found difficult to preserve the lactic acid ferment for a long time in a living condition. Amongst the ferments which have been isolated from Egyptian ' leben ' by MM. Rist and Khoury[1] there is one which is extremely delicate.

[1] *Annales de l'Institut Pasteur*, 1902, p. 71.

When it is inoculated deep in a nutritive medium, it dies in a few days, death, without doubt, being due to the lactic acid produced by the microbe from the sugar and not neutralised. As this transformation of sugar into lactic acid is a fundamental property of the microbe, depending on its constitution, the arrest of the fermentation and the death of the ferment in these definite conditions can be interpreted only as natural death due to auto-intoxication, that is to say to poisoning by a product of the physiological activity of the microbe itself. As death takes place at a time when the medium still contains enough sugar for the nutrition of the microbe, it is certain that it cannot be the result of exhaustion. This case of the lactic acid ferment is not unique. The microbe which produces butyric acid is also interfered with by the acid it secretes. M. G. Bertrand, who has examined carefully the microbe which produces fermentation in sorbose (sugar extracted from fruit of the service-tree) (*Sorbus domestica*) has informed me that this fermentation, too, ceases under the influence of the secretions of the microbes, and that the microbes undergo natural death at a time when the medium is far from exhausted of the nutritive material. The yeast which produces alcohol is also interfered with by an excess of alcohol, and as soon as a certain limit of alcoholic strength has been reached, fermentation stops. When the yeast is grown in media rich in nitrogen and poor in sugar, the plant takes the nitrogenous material and produces salts of ammonia. These alkalies damage the yeast and cause its death by auto-intoxication.[1]

In the examples that I have given, natural death was a result of the activity of the microbes, and was in correlation with their organisation. Such death can be

[1] Duclaux, *Microbiologie*, vol. iii, 1900, p. 460.

NATURAL DEATH AMONG PLANTS

avoided by changing the external conditions, and, if the acids or alkalies produced by these bacteria are neutralised, the bacteria survive. The facts are in harmony with those that I described in the case of the higher plants. By preventing the ripening of seed, the life of many annual plants may be preserved and the plants changed to biennials or perennials. In such cases death, although the result of the constitution of the plant, may be postponed.

We may ask then if the natural death of higher plants, usually attributed to exhaustion, cannot be explained more simply as the result of poisons produced in their metabolism. Many plants produce poisons which are fatal to animals and man. May they not also produce substances fatal to themselves? There is nothing improbable in the supposition that some of the poisons may develop when the seeds are ripening. By preventing the latter process, the ripening of the whole organism may also be prevented. Such a theory would explain the many cases of natural death which occur whilst the cell is far from having reached exhaustion. The equally numerous cases of partial death, such as that of flowers, whilst the same stem is still producing other flowers (*e.g.* geraniums) would be explained by a local action of the poisons not strong enough to kill the whole plant.

I must insist that this theory, that natural death of the higher plants, is the result of auto-intoxication, is a mere hypothesis which future investigations may disprove. If, however, it comes to be confirmed, it would explain the coincidence of death and fructification more simply than the hypothesis of predestination.

The higher plants may be subjects of auto-intoxication in the same fashion as bacteria and yeasts. If these poisons were produced before the ripening of the seeds, the plants would remain sterile, leaving no descendants, so that the race would become extinct. The production of poisons at the time of fructification would not interfere with the succession of generations, and the race would be preserved. As the poisoning is not necessary, it is easy to understand why many plants survive seeding and escape natural death. The Dragon-tree, baobab, and the cedars, which I spoke of earlier, would be examples of such escape.

Although the existence of auto-intoxication in the higher plants is still only a hypothesis, the natural death of bacteria and yeasts by poisons which they themselves produce is an ascertained fact.

In the plant world, therefore, there are examples of natural death (bacteria and yeasts) due to auto-intoxication, and there are other cases where high or low plants escape natural death.

II

NATURAL DEATH IN THE ANIMAL WORLD

Different origins of natural death in animals—Examples of natural death associated with violent acts—Examples of natural death in animals without digestive organs—Natural death in the two sexes—Hypothesis as to the cause of natural death in animals

THE cases of natural death amongst animals differ from those found in the vegetable world by their greater variety and complexity. As M. Massart has shown for plants, so also natural death must have become established independently in different groups of animals. In some cases, the characters presented are strange and almost paradoxical.

It is usual to contrast natural death with violent death on account of the difference between the two. None the less, natural death may occur in the animal kingdom, that is to say death resulting directly from the constitution, and yet in intimate association with violent acts. I will give some examples.

Small, helmet-shaped organisms, transparent and graceful, are common on the surface of the sea. These have been described by zoologists under the name *Pilidium*. The organisation is simple. The body wall is a delicate pellicle, through which, on the lower surface, a mouth leads into a capacious stomach. Continual movements of waving cilia direct small particles of food through the mouth to the digestive stomach. As there are no organs of reproduction, it was assumed that these creatures were not adults, but floating larvæ of some marine animal, and, after a good deal of trouble, it was found that the Pilidia were the young stages of ribbon-shaped worms of the group of Nemertines. At a definite stage in the life-history, a fœtus begins to develop round about the stomach of the Pilidium, and eventually completely encloses it and detaches it by violent muscular contractions. The end of the story is that the fœtus abandons the body of the Pilidium carrying off with it the stomach, an organ necessary to the maintenance of life. The remnant of the Pilidium swims about in the sea-water, but soon dies as the result of the mortal wound caused by the removal of the digestive organs.

The act by which the Nemertine separates from its mother is violent, and yet the death of the Pilidium must be regarded as natural. It is the result of agencies within the body and not, as in most cases of accidental death, of violence from without.

The group of Nematode worms contains many common intestinal parasites of man, such as *Ascaris, Trichina, Trichocephalus, Oxyuris*, &c., but also others that live free in soil or water or in such fluids as vinegar. They are protected by a strong cuticle, and some of them are viviparous, that is to say, instead of laying eggs they give birth to young worms already well grown and capable of independent activity. Amongst the human Nematode parasites, the *Trichinæ* give birth to swarms of small larvæ which easily escape from the body of the mother by the female generative aperture. In the case of some free-living Nematodes, however, the female aperture is too small to give passage to the rather stout larvæ. More than forty years ago, when I was investigating the life-history[1] of one of these Nematodes (*Diplogaster tridentatus*) I was struck by the fact that the larvæ could leave the body of the mother only by violence and after they had devoured most of its substance. These larvæ develop from eggs produced within the maternal body. As the external reproductive aperture of the female is minute, the larvæ cannot escape through it, but wander amongst the tissues tearing and absorbing them. The mother soon dies, and although her death is violent, it must be included in the category of natural death.

From the teleological point of view it might be said that Pilidium and Diplogaster cease to live because they have fulfilled their function of giving rise to a Nemertine or young Nematodes. Their natural death would thus be predestined. There is no ground for such an interpretation. On the other hand, it is certain that this death, coming after the birth of the new generation, is in no way against the preservation of the species in which the extraordinary natural death by violence occurs. If the female orifice of Diplogaster were slightly larger, the larvæ would emerge without difficulty and without causing the death of the mother which none the less would have fulfilled her purpose.

All the cases of natural death amongst animals are not so brutal as those of the Pilidium and the Nemertine worms. In many instances the death is peaceful. As very frequently it is difficult to establish definitely that the death is natural, I shall select clear cases.

Animals are occasionally found which are devoid of some organ necessary for prolonged life. The absence of a

[1] *Archiv. für Anatomie und Physiologie*, 1864.

digestive tract in an animal that lives in an environment rich in dissolved nutritive material (as for instance tapeworms living in the intestinal tract) is not surprising. But when creatures of the sea or of fresh water have no digestive tract, their life can be maintained only at the expense of nutritive material stored within them during embryonic life. The death which comes eventually is truly natural. The best cases, that is to say those which can be studied most completely, of such natural death occur amongst the Rotifera. These are minute creatures of fresh or sea water, at one time confused with the Infusoria, but possessed of a much more complex organisation. They have a well-developed digestive tube, organs of excretion, nervous system, and organs of sense. The animals are diœcious; in each species both males and females exist. Whilst the females have the complete structure of the species, the males are much reduced, and are devoid of a digestive canal. The cuticle is fairly stout, and they are unable to absorb dissolved nutriment through it; as they have no organs of digestion, their life must be short.

To study in detail the life and death of these creatures, I selected a species sent to me by M. Haffkine. So far as I can judge, the species in question is a hitherto unknown member of the genus *Pleurotrocha,* and I propose for it the name *Pleurotrocha haffkini.* This rotifer is convenient to study as it thrives in vessels containing fresh-water to which some bread-crumb has been added (in the proportion of a gram of bread to 500 grams of water).

The sexes of the little rotifer can be distinguished from the earliest age, for eggs that are to become females are much larger than those from which males develop. It is easy to isolate the male eggs and to follow the life-history up to the moment of natural death. The whole course of life from the laying of the egg until death lasts only about three days, and is probably the shortest duration of life in the animal kingdom. Although some Ephemeridæ live only a few hours in the adult state, their total life-cycle is much longer than that of the rotifers, as the larval stages last for months or even for years.

The little males (Fig. 16) begin to swim soon after hatching, the wheel-apparatus and the musculature being vigorous. They seek out the females, as their reproductive organs are mature almost at the moment of hatching. The transparent body, which is devoid of digestive ap-

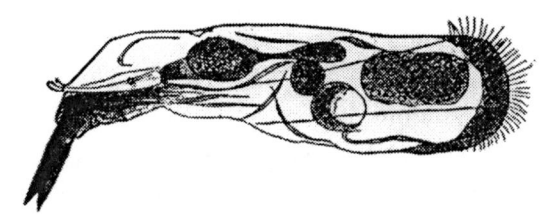

FIG. 16.—Male *Pleurotrocha haffkini*.

paratus, swarms with mobile spermatozoa. As soon as the male has seized a female, he discharges the contents of his body. It might be supposed that such an evacuation would cause a violent perturbation of the system leading to the death of the organism. There is no question of this however. The males are able to live for twenty-four hours after having accomplished their function, and the period represents a third of their total duration of life. Moreover, I have isolated males from females without any prolongation of their lives. In one experiment, I isolated two males and placed a third in company with two females. It was the third specimen that lived longest.

The natural death of the males is foreshadowed by a weakening of the movements; although the muscles and cilia remain mobile, the whole animal moves only spasmodically; sometimes the muscles of the head contract, sometimes those of the tail, but no locomotion occurs. Occasionally there is a violent effort of ciliary motion as if the attempt were being made to overcome the immobility of the body. Such a condition lasts for several hours and is followed by death. The spermatozoa inside the body retain activity last of all.

Towards the crisis, bacteria, which abound in the medium occupied by the rotifers, begin to attack the males. Some cluster round the head, others round the tail, although none of them can effect entrance to the body. The death of the males cannot be attributed to microbial infection, but comes from some intrinsic cause.

Is it inanition that is the cause of death? I do not think so, because up to the time of death the tissues appear to be unmodified. In the case of the females I have sometimes seen phenomena of inanition. In old and exhausted cultures the starved females become thin, flattened and quite transparent, and the tissues lose their granular appearance. No such changes are visible in the dying males, the tissues of which, on the contrary, retain a normal aspect.

The most probable explanation is that death comes from poisoning by the secretions of the tissues themselves. The large size of the organs of excretion indicates that in the course of metabolism waste matter is produced some of which is got rid of. If, after a time, the secretions are insufficiently eliminated, the tissues must be poisoned. As death is preceded by a spasm of uncoordinated movement, it appears as if the fatal intoxication of the males affected the nervous system first. The vibrating cilia and the muscles are attacked later.

There can be no doubt but that the death of these male

NATURAL DEATH IN ANIMAL WORLD

rotifers is natural in the fullest sense. The females, however, although they are provided with complete digestive organs, do not escape a similar fate. Their life is longer and more complex than that of the males, and so is subject to many more chances. The females therefore may come to die from starvation or from other external, accidental causes. But, if they are kept in favourable conditions, they may live for about fifteen days, towards the end of which they die naturally, exhibiting the symptoms that I have described in the case of the males (Fig. 17).

Rotifers are not the only animals which undergo natural death in a fashion quite unlike the violent end of Pilidium

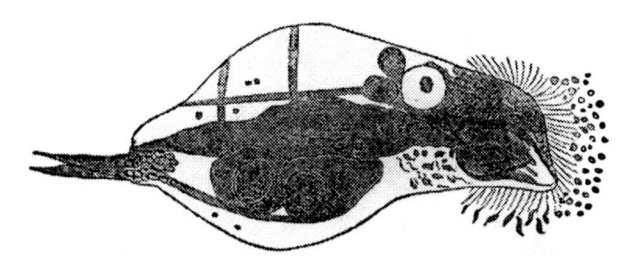

FIG. 17.—Female *Pleurotrocha haffkini*, which has died a natural death.

and Diplogaster. There are other cases amongst invertebrates, but I shall limit myself to describing one that is well ascertained.

More than fifty years ago, Dana, the American naturalist, discovered a pelagic marine creature with characters so curious that he gave to it the name *Monstrilla*. It is a little crustacean akin to the *Cyclops* of lakes. But although the latter is endowed with the organs necessary to capture and digest food, *Monstrilla* has neither organs of prehension nor a digestive canal. It is a highly muscular animal with organs of sense and reproduction and a nervous system; but it is devoid of apparatus for prolonging life by nutrition. *Monstrilla* therefore is a creature doomed to natural death.

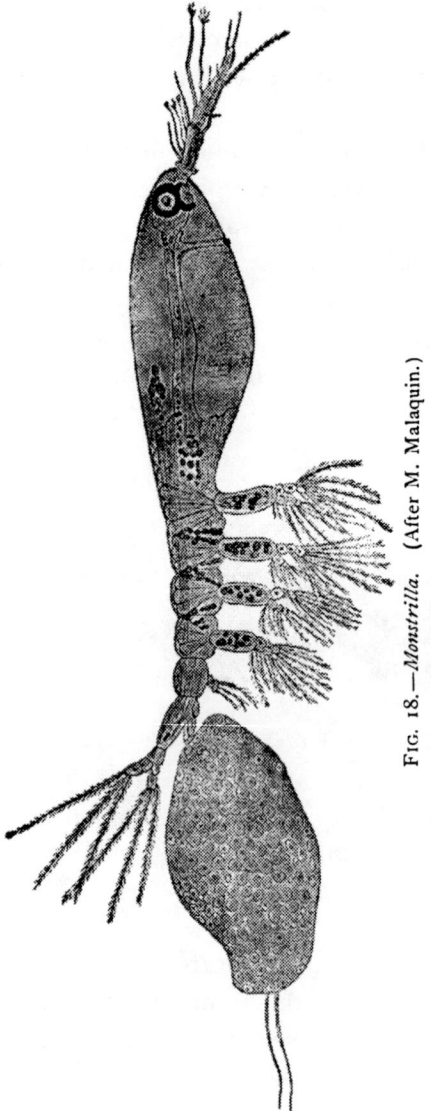

The detailed observations of M. Malaquin[1] have supplied full information regarding this strange life-history. *Monstrilla* passes a portion of its life as a parasite on Annelid worms. In that stage it accumulates the necessary material for the growth of the sexual products (ova and spermatozoa) and for free life in the sea whilst the young are developing. It is not only the males which have no digestive apparatus. The females also lack it, which is the more surprising as they carry about the eggs attached to the body (as is done by many other Crustacea, such as crayfish and lobsters) until the young are ready to hatch (Fig. 18). M. Malaquin thinks that the Monstrillas die of starvation.

FIG. 18.—*Monstrilla*. (After M. Malaquin.)

[1] *Archives de Zoologie expérimentale*, 1901, vol. ix, p. 81.

"As they are without a digestive tube or organs of prehension or mastication," M. Malaquin says (p. 192), "the Monstrillas, which have no means of nutrition, are doomed to death from inanition after a short pelagic life. This is a logical inference from their structure."

In support of his view, M. Malaquin states that before death the tissues and organs show plain signs of degeneration.

"The eyes first show traces of degeneration. The pigment spreads and disappears little by little and then the visual elements fade out."

"Finally, individuals, usually females, show complete degeneration. A female taken in a fine-meshed net showed no trace of organs in the head; the eyes, the brain and the intestinal tract had disappeared almost completely. The antennæ were reduced to stumps consisting of the lowest joint and a portion of the second. These were clear indications of the senility that precedes death" (p. 194).

Such evidence not only supports the hypothesis that the natural death of Monstrilla is due to inanition, but is opposed to a similar interpretation being applied to the case of male rotifers, in which death is not preceded by wasting of the organs. The death of some insects, which comes rapidly after the adult stage has been reached, cannot readily be attributed to starvation. In the strange butterflies known as psychids (*Solenobia*) some of the females lay eggs without having been fertilised,[1] and their life in the adult condition lasts only a day. On the other hand, other females of the same butterfly are fertilised before laying their eggs and in this case survive for more than a week although they take no food. The rapid death of the first-mentioned set cannot be attributed to inanition.

[1] Observations of Dr. Speyer, quoted by Weismann.

In some Ephemeridæ, which supply good cases of natural death, the end comes after a few hours of adult life without any sign of degeneration of the organs. As in others (*Chloë*), life lasts for several days without food having been taken, it is clear that inanition is not the cause of the swift arrival of death in the first set. It is much more probable that the natural death is due to an auto-intoxication which takes effect at different intervals of time in different circumstances.[1]

In the higher animals such as vertebrates the conditions are less favourable than in the case of insects for the investigation of the causes of natural death. Vertebrates have always well-developed organs of digestion and so live a relatively longer time and encounter a greater number of chances of accident, with the result that in most cases death comes from external accidental causes. Vertebrates usually perish from hunger or cold, or are devoured by their enemies or killed by the attacks of parasites or diseases. There remains only the human race amongst the more highly developed animals, in which to study the onset of natural death. And in the human race cases which may be designated as natural are extremely rare.

[1] See *The Nature of Man.*

III

NATURAL DEATH AMONGST HUMAN BEINGS

Natural death in the aged—Analogy of natural death and sleep—Theories of sleep—Ponogenes—The instinct of sleep—The instinct of natural death—Replies to critics—Agreeable sensation at the approach of death

THE death of old people, which has often been described as natural death, is in most cases due to infectious diseases, particularly pneumonia (which is extremely dangerous) or to attacks of apoplexy. True natural death must be very rare in the human race. Demange[1] has described it as follows:—"Arrived at extreme old age, and still preserving the last flickers of an expiring intelligence, the old man feels weakness gaining on him from day to day. His limbs refuse to obey his will, the skin becomes insensitive, dry, and cold; the extremities lose their warmth; the face is thin; the eyes hollow and the sight weak; speech dies out on his lips which remain open; life quits the old man from the circumference towards the centre; breathing grows laboured, and at last the heart stops beating. The old man passes away quietly, seeming to fall asleep for the last time." Such is the course of what properly speaking is natural death.

The natural death of human beings cannot be regarded as due to exhaustion from reproduction or from inanition,

[1] *Étude clinique sur la vieillesse*, Paris, 1886, p. 145.

as in the case of *Monstrilla*. It is much more likely that it is due to an auto-intoxication of the organism. The close analogy between natural death and sleep supports this view, as it is very probable that sleep is due to poisoning by the products of organic activity.

It is more than fifty years since sleep was explained as the result of auto-intoxication. Obersteiner, Binz, Preyer, and Errera are among the competent men of science who have taken this view. The first two attributed sleep to an accumulation in the brain of the products of exhaustion which are carried away by the blood during repose. The attempt has been made even to discover the nature of these narcotic substances. Some investigators think that an acid, produced during the activity of the organs, is stored up in quantities that cannot be tolerated. During sleep, the organism gets rid of this excess of acid.

Preyer[1] tried to put the problem upon a more exact basis by the theory that the activity of all the organs gives rise to substances which he called *ponogenes* and which he regarded as producing the sensation of fatigue. According to him these substances accumulate during the waking hours, and are destroyed by oxidation during sleep. Preyer thinks that lactic acid is the most important of the ponogenes, and lays stress on its narcotic effect. If his theory were correct, there would be a remarkable analogy between the auto-intoxication by lactic acid in the cases of man and animals, and the case of bacteria which produce the same acid and the fermenting activity of which is arrested as the acid accumulates. Just as sleep may be transformed to natural death, so also the arrest of lactic fermentation may be followed by the death of the bacteria which form the acid.

[1] *Revue scientifique*, 1877, p. 1173.

So far, however, there has been no confirmation of Preyer's theory. Errera[1] has brought forward against it another theory according to which the cause of sleep is not acid products, but certain alkaline substances described by M. Armand Gautier under the name of *leucomaines.* Gautier laid down that these substances act on the nervous centres and produce fatigue and sleepiness. According to Errera they might very well be the cause of sleep, as that comes on at a time when there is the greatest accumulation of these leucomaines in the body. He thinks that their action in producing sleep is a direct intoxication of the nerve centres. During sleep they are removed, and the disturbance which was produced in the organism is arrested.

If it were possible to accept Errera's theory, a kind of analogy could be established between sleep and natural death on the one hand, and the arrest of development and death of yeast grown in nitrogenous media on the other hand, because in the latter case the poisoning is produced by an alkaline salt of ammonia. It must be confessed, however, that the actual state of our knowledge does not allow of a definite view of the real mechanism of the sleep-producing intoxication. Our ideas regarding leucomaines in general are still incomplete, and, recently, one of them, *adrenaline,* the product of the supra-renal capsules, has been investigated. Adrenaline is an alkaloid[2] which is produced in the supra-renal bodies and is discharged into the blood. It has the power of contracting arteries strongly, and has been used to control blood-pressure. When it is given in large quantities or in frequent doses, it acts as a true poison, whilst, in small doses, it produces anæmia of the organs and has a special influence on the nervous

[1] *Revue scientifique,* 1887, 2nd part, p. 105.
[2] Gabriel Bertrand, *Annales de l'Institut Pasteur,* 1904, p. 672.

centres. Dr. Zeigan[1] has shown that a milligramme of adrenaline, mixed with five grammes of normal salt solution injected into the brain of cats, produces a soporific action. "About a minute after the injection, the animal appears to be plunged into deep sleep which lasts from 30 to 50 minutes. During this time, the sensitiveness of the animal has completely ceased throughout the body, and for some time after that it is much decreased. When they awake the animals seem to have been drunk with sleep for some time." Sleep is generally associated with anæmia of the brain, and as adrenaline can actually produce such anæmia, it might be supposed that this narcotic substance is the most important of the organic products which give rise to sleep. Against this hypothesis, however, some weight must be given to recent investigations on fatigue and its causes.

Each stage in the advance of knowledge has had its influence on the study of the interesting and complex problem of sleep. When it was thought that alkaloids (ptomaines) were of great importance in infectious diseases, it was attempted to explain sleep as due to the action of similar bodies. Now, when we believe that in such diseases the chief part is played by poisons of extremely complex chemical composition, the attempt is made to explain fatigue and sleep by similar bodies.

Weichardt[2] has recently made the best known investigations in this direction. This young man maintains with ardour the view that during the activity of organs there is an accumulation of special materials which are neither organic acids nor leucomaines, but which are much more like the toxic products of pathogenic bacteria.

[1] *Therapeutische Monatshefte*, 1904, p. 193.
[2] *Münchener medicinische Wochenschrift*, 1904, No. 1; *Verhandlungen der physiologischen Gesellschaft zu Berlin*, Dec. 5th, 1904.

NATURAL DEATH

Weichardt made animals in his laboratory go through fatiguing movements for hours and then killed them. The extract from muscles of such animals had a powerful toxic effect when it was injected into normal animals, producing lassitude and sometimes death within 20 to 40 hours. As all attempts to determine the exact chemical nature of this fatigue-producing substance were baffled, it is impossible to get an exact account of it. Amongst its properties there is one of great interest. When it has passed into the circulation of normal animals in quantities insufficient to produce death, it excites the formation of an anti-toxin in the same way as a poison of diphtheria stimulates the production of a diphtheria anti-toxin.

When Weichardt injected into animals a mixture of the poison which produces fatigue with small doses of the serum antidote, no results followed. The neutralising effect of the antidote was apparent even when it was introduced by the mouth. Towards the end of his investigations, Weichardt supposed that it would be possible to obtain a material that would prevent fatigue.

Although it is still impossible to specify exactly the nature of the substances which accumulate during the activity of organs and which produce fatigue and sleep, it is becoming more and more probable that such substances exist, and that sleep is really an auto-intoxication of the organism. So far, such a theory has not been shaken by any argument. Recently M. E. Claparède,[1] a psychologist of Geneva, has argued against the current theory of sleep. He thinks that it is contradicted by the fact that new-born infants sleep a great deal, whilst very old people sleep very little. This fact, however, can readily be ex-

[1] *Archives des sciences physiques et naturelles*, Geneva, March, 1905, vol. xvii ; *Archives de physiologie*, vol. iv, p. 245.

plained by the greater sensibility of the nerve centres of infants, as shown with regard to many harmful agencies. The other objections of Claparède, such as the fact that sleepiness is induced by exercise in the open air, or that excess of sleep itself produces sleepiness, are not really incompatible with the theory of auto-intoxication. They are facts of secondary importance probably depending on some complication which the present state of our knowledge makes it difficult to indicate exactly. The insomnia of neurasthenia, which Claparède brings forward as another objection, can readily be explained as due to hyperæsthesia of the nervous tissues which lose part of their sensitiveness to poisons.

On the other hand, there are many well established facts in agreement with the theory of auto-intoxication. Leaving out of the question sleep induced by narcotics, I may mention in this connection the so-called " sleeping sickness." It has been proved that this disease is caused by a microscopic parasite, the *Trypanosoma gambiense* of Dutton, which develops in the blood and spreads to the liquid of the membranes surrounding the central nervous system. One of the most typical symptoms of the advanced stages of this disease is continual drowsiness. " The drowsiness increases progressively, and the habitual attitude becomes characteristic; the head is bent on the breast; the eyelids are closed; in earlier stages the invalid can be aroused easily, but, after a time, incurable attacks of sleep overcome the patient in all circumstances, but especially after meals. These fits of sleepiness become longer and deeper, until they reach a comatose condition from which it is almost impossible to arouse the patient."[1] The total

[1] Laveran and Mesnil, *Trypanosomes et Trypanosomiases*, Paris, 1904, p. 328.

result of medical knowledge of this disease is that it is impossible to doubt that the sleepiness is due to intoxication produced by the poison of the trypanosome.

Claparède has opposed what he calls an "instinctive" theory to the toxic theory of sleep. According to this theory, sleep is the manifestation of an instinct "the object of which is to arrest activity; we do not sleep because we are intoxicated or exhausted, but to prevent ourselves from falling into such a condition." However, in order to bring this narcotic instinct into play, certain conditions are necessary, one of which certainly would be the intoxication of the nerve centres. M. Claparède supposes that sleep is an active phenomenon, induced when waste matter begins to accumulate in the organism. "To bring about sleep, the nerve centres must be influenced by waste matter, and this influence can readily be regarded as a kind of intoxication."

Hunger is an instinctive sensation as much as sleepiness, but it does not appear until our tissues are in a condition of exhaustion, the exact nature of which cannot as yet be indicated. There is no real contradiction between the toxic and instinctive theories of sleep. The two theories represent different sides of a special condition of the organism.

The analogy between sleep and natural death is in favour of the supposition that the latter, also, is due to an intoxication much more profound and serious than that which results in sleep. Therefore, as natural death in human beings has been studied only very superficially, it is impossible to do more than frame theories regarding it.

It would be natural if, just as in sleep there is an instinctive desire for rest, so also the natural death of man were preceded by an instinctive wish for it. As I have already discussed this subject in the "Nature of Man" (chap. xi)

I need not deal with it at length here. I should like, however, to add some information which I have recently obtained.

The most striking fact in favour of the existence of the instinct for natural death in man appears to me to have been related by Tokarsky in regard to an old woman. While Tokarsky was alive I asked one of his friends to obtain for me further details of this very interesting case. Unfortunately Tokarsky could add nothing to what he had already published in his article. I think that I have discovered the source of his information. In his famous book on the *Physiology of Taste*[1] Brillat-Savarin relates as follows:—" A great-aunt of mine died at the age of 93. Although she had been confined to bed for some time her faculties were still well preserved, and the only evidence of her condition was the decrease in appetite and weakening of her voice. She had always been very friendly to me, and once when I was at her bedside, ready to tend her affectionately, although that did not hinder me from seeing her with the philosophical eye that I always turned on everything about me, 'Is it you, my nephew?' she said in her feeble voice. 'Yes, Aunt, I am here at your service, and I think you will do very well to take a drop of this good old wine.' 'Give it me, my dear; I can always take a little wine.' I made ready at once, and gently supporting her, gave her half a glass of my best wine. She brightened up at once, and turning on me her eyes which used to be so beautiful, said: 'Thank you very much for this last kindness; if you ever reach my age you will find that one wants to die just as one wants to sleep.' These were her last words, and in half an hour she fell into her last sleep." The details make it certain that this was

[1] Paris, 1834, 4th edition, vol. ii, p. 118.

a case of the instinct of natural death. The instinct showed itself at an age not very great in the case of a woman who had preserved her mental faculties. Generally, however, it seems not to appear till much later, for old men usually exhibit a keen wish to live.

It is a well-known saying that the longer a man has lived the more he wishes to live. Charles Renouvier,[1] a French philosopher who died a few years ago, has left a definite proof of the truth of the saying. When he was eighty-eight years old, and knew that he was dying, he recorded his impressions in his last days. Let me quote from what he wrote four days before his death. " I have no illusions about my condition; I know quite well that I am going to die, perhaps in a week, perhaps in a fortnight. And I have still so much to say on my subject." "At my age I have no longer the right to hope: my days are numbered, and perhaps my hours. I must resign myself." " I do not die without regrets. I regret that I cannot foresee in any way the fate of my views." "And I am leaving the world before I have said my last word. A man always dies before he has finished his work, and that is the saddest of the sorrows of life." " But that is not the whole trouble, when a man is old, very old, and accustomed to life, it is very difficult to die. I think that young men accept the idea of dying more easily, perhaps more willingly than old men. When one is more than eighty years old, one is cowardly and shrinks from death. And when one knows and can no longer doubt that death is coming near, deep bitterness falls on the soul." " I have faced the question from all sides in the last few days; I turn the one idea over in my mind; I *know* that I am going to die, but I cannot *persuade* myself that I am going to die. It is not the

[1] *Revue de métaphysique et de morale*, March, 1904.

philosopher in me that protests. The philosopher does not fear death; it is the *old man*. The old man has not the courage to submit, and yet I have to submit to the inevitable."

I know a lady, a hundred and two years old, who is so oppressed by the idea of death, that those about her have to conceal from her the death of any of her acquaintances. Mde. Robineau, however, when between one hundred and four and one hundred and five years old, became quite indifferent to the close approach of her own death. She often expressed a wish for it, thinking herself useless in the world.

M. Yves Delage[1] in an analysis of my "Nature of Man" doubted the existence of an instinct for death. "Animals," said he, "cannot have the instinct for death, because they do not know of death. In their case, we must consider that what happens is an apathy tending to the abolition of the sense of self-preservation. In man, the knowledge of death implies that the indifference to its approach cannot be an instinct." "There may be developed, at the end of life, a special state of mind which accepts death with indifference or with pleasure, but such a state cannot be designated as an instinct." M. Delage, however, does not suggest what the state of mind in question is to be called. As the aunt of Brillat-Savarin compared her sensations just before death with the desire to sleep, and as this desire is an instinctive manifestation, I think that the cheerful acquiescence in death, exhibited by extremely old people, is also a kind of instinct. However, the important matter is that the sentiment exists, and not what we are to call it. M. Delage is far from denying its existence.

[1] *Année biologique*, vol. vii, p. 595.

Dr. Cancalon,[1] another of my critics, cannot admit the existence of an instinct of death, "because of the theory of evolution. Of what good would it have been, as M. Metchnikoff tells us that natural death is very rare; how could it have been transmitted, as it comes into existence long after the age of reproduction, and how could it have aided the survival of the species? If its existence were proved as the result of biological evolution, it would be a contradiction of adaptation and an argument in favour of final causes." I cannot agree in any way with these opinions. In the first place, it is well known that men and animals have many harmful instincts that do not tend to the survival of the species. I need recall only the disharmonic instincts which I described in the "Nature of Man," such as the anomalies of the sexual instinct, the instinct which drives parents to devour their young or which attracts insects to flames. The instinct of natural death is far from being harmful, and may even have many advantages. If men were convinced that the end of life were natural death accompanied by a special instinct like that of the need for sleep, one of the greatest sources of pessimism would disappear. Now pessimism is the cause of the voluntary death of a certain number of people and of many others refraining from reproduction. The instinct of natural death would contribute to the maintenance of the life of the individual and of the species. On the other hand, there is no difficulty in admitting the existence of instincts hostile to the preservation of the species, especially in the case of man, in whom individualism has reached its highest development. As man is the only animal with a definite notion of death, there is nothing extraordinary if it is in man that the instinctive wish for

[1] *Revue occidentale*, July 1st, 1904, vol. xxx, p. 87.

death develops. M. Cancalon denies the possibility that death can be pleasant, as it is the arrest of the physiological functions; but as sleep and syncope are often preceded by very pleasant sensations, why may not this also happen in natural death? Several facts prove it beyond dispute. It is even probable that the approach of natural death is one of the most pleasant sensations that can exist.

It is indubitable that in a large number of cases of death, the cessation of life is associated with very painful sensations. One has only to see the horror shown in the faces of many dying people to be convinced of this, but there are diseases and serious accidents in which the approach of death does not arouse sorrowful sensations. I myself, in a crisis of intermittent fever, in which the temperature descended in a very short time from about 106° Fahr. to below normal, experienced a feeling of extraordinary weakness, certainly like that at the approach of death. This sensation was much more pleasant than painful. In two cases of serious morphia poisoning, my sensations were more agreeable; I felt a pleasant weakness, associated with a sensation of lightness of the body, as if I were floating in the air.

Those who have noted the sensations of persons rescued from death have related similar facts. Prof. Heim, of Zurich, has described a fall in the mountains which nearly killed him, as well as several similar accidents to Alpine tourists. In all these cases he states that there was a sensation of pleasure.[1] Dr. Sollier has told of a young woman addicted to morphia, who had been convinced that she was at the point of death. On recovering from a most serious attack of syncope, from which she was restored only by giving another dose of morphia, she cried: "I seem to

[1] Egger, "*Le moi des mourants*," Revue philosophique, 1896, i, p. 27.

come from far away; how happy I was!" Another of Dr. Sollier's patients, a lady who had an attack of peritonitis from which she expected to die, felt herself "suffused with a feeling of well-being, or rather the absence of all pain." In a third case of Dr. Sollier, a young woman suffering from puerperal fever, feeling herself at the point of death, had a similar sensation "of physical well-being and of detachment from everything."[1]

As a sensation of happiness occurs even in cases of pathological death, it is much more likely to occur in natural death. If natural death be preceded by the loss of the instinct of life and by the acquisition of a new instinct, it would be the best possible end compatible with the real organisation of human nature.

I do not pretend to give the reader a finished study on natural death. This chapter of Thanatology, the science of death, only opens the subject; but it is already apparent that study of the circumstances of natural death in plants, in the animal world, and in human beings, may give facts of the highest interest to science and humanity.

[1] *Ibid.*, pp. 303-307 ; v. also *Bulletin de l'Institut général phycholog.*, 1903, p. 29.

PART IV

SHOULD WE TRY TO PROLONG HUMAN LIFE?

I

THE BENEFIT TO HUMANITY

Complaints of the shortness of our life—Theory of " medical selection " as a cause of degeneration of the race—Utility of prolonging human life

ALTHOUGH the duration of the life of man is one of the longest amongst mammals, men find it too short. From the remotest times the shortness of life has been complained of, and there have been many attempts to prolong it. Man has not been satisfied with a duration of life notably greater than that of his nearest relatives, and has wished to live at least as long as reptiles.

In antiquity, Hippocrates and Aristotle thought that human life was too short, and Theophrastus, although he died at an advanced age (he lived probably seventy-five years) lamented when he was dying " that nature had given to deer and to crows a life so long and so useless, and to man only one that was often very short." [1]

Seneca (*De brevitate vitæ*) and later, in the 18th century, Haller, strove in vain against such complaints, which have lasted until our own days. Whilst animals have no more

[1] Cicero, *Tusculanes*, chap. xxviii.

THE BENEFIT TO HUMANITY 133

than an instinctive fear of danger, and cling to life without knowing what death is, men have acquired an exact idea of death, and their knowledge increases their desire to live.

Ought we to listen to the cry of humanity that life is too short and that it would be well to prolong it? Would it really be for the good of the human race to extend the duration of the life of man beyond its present limits? Already it is complained that the burden of supporting old people is too heavy, and statesmen are perturbed by the enormous expense which will be entailed by State support of the aged. In France, in a population of about 38 millions, there are two millions (1,912,153) who have reached the age of 70, that is to say, about five per cent. of the total. The support of these old people absorbs a sum of nearly £6,000,000 per annum.[1] However generous may be the views of the members of the French Parliament, many of them hesitate at the idea of so great a burden. Without doubt, men say, the cost of maintaining the aged will become still heavier if the duration of life is to be prolonged. If old people are to live longer, the resources of the young will be reduced.

If the question were merely one of prolonging the life of old people without modifying old age itself, such considerations would be justified. It must be understood, however, that the prolongation of life would be associated with the preservation of intelligence and of the power to work. In the earlier parts of this book I have given many examples which show the possibility of useful work being done by persons of advanced years. When we have reduced or abolished such causes of precocious senility as intemperance and disease, it will no longer be necessary to give pensions

[1] Rapport de M. Bienvenu-Martin à la Chambre des députés, Paris, 1903.

at the age of sixty or seventy years. The cost of supporting the old, instead of increasing, will diminish progressively.

If attainment of the normal duration of life, which is much greater than the average life to-day, were to over-populate the earth, a very remote possibility, this could be remedied by lowering the birth-rate. Even at the present time, while the earth is far from being too quickly peopled, artificial limitation of the birth-rate takes place perhaps to an unnecessary extent.

It has long been a charge against medicine and hygiene that they tend to weaken the human race. By scientific means unhealthy people, or those with inherited blemishes, have been preserved so that they can give birth to weak offspring. If natural selection were allowed free play, such individuals would perish and make room for others, stronger and better able to live. Haeckel has given the name "medical selection" to this process under which humanity degenerates because of the influence of medical science.

It is clear that a valuable existence of great service to humanity is compatible with a feeble constitution and precarious health. Amongst tuberculous people, those with inherited or acquired syphilis, and those with a constitution unbalanced in other ways, that is to say, amongst so-called degenerates, there have been individuals who have had a large share in the advance of the human race. I need only instance the names of Fresnel, Leopardi, Weber, Schumann and Chopin. It does not follow that we ought to cherish diseases and leave to natural selection the duty of preserving the individuals which can resist them. On the other hand, it is indispensable to try to blot out the diseases themselves, and, in particular, the evils of old age, by the methods of hygiene and therapeutics. The theory of medical selection must be given up as contrary to the good of the human race. We must use all our endeavours to allow men to complete their normal course of life, and to make it possible for old men to play their parts as advisers and judges, endowed with their long experience of life.

To the question propounded at the beginning of this section of my book, I can make only one answer: Yes, it is useful to prolong human life.

II

SUGGESTIONS FOR THE PROLONGATION OF LIFE

Ancient methods of prolonging human life—Gerokomy—The "immortality draught" of the Taoists—Brown-Séquard's method—The spermine of Poehl—Dr. Weber's precepts—Increased duration of life in historical times—Hygienic maxims—Decrease in cutaneous cancer

MEN of all times have attempted all manner of devices to bring about an increase of years, although they have not considered the problem in its general bearing.

In Biblical times it was believed that contact with young girls would rejuvenate and prolong the life of feeble old men. In the first Book of Kings it is related as follows:—

"Now King David was old and stricken in years; and they covered him with clothes, but he gat no heat.

"Wherefore his servants said unto him, Let there be sought for my Lord the king a young virgin; let her stand before the king and let her cherish him, and let her lie in thy bosom, that my lord the king may get heat" (Kings I., chap. i.).

This device, afterwards called *gerokomy*, was employed by the Greeks and Romans, and has had followers in modern times. Boerhave, the famous Dutch physician (1668—1738), "recommended an old burgomaster of Amsterdam to lie between two young girls, assuring him that he would thus recover strength and spirits." After quoting this, Hufeland, the well-known author of "Macro-

SUGGESTIONS FOR PROLONGING LIFE 137

biotique" in the eighteenth century, made the following reflection :—"If it be remembered how the exhalations from newly opened animals stimulate paralysed limbs, and how the application of living animals soothes a violent pain, we cannot refuse our approval to the method."[1]

Cohausen, a doctor of the eighteenth century, published a treatise on a Roman, Hermippus, who had died aged a hundred and fifteen years. He had been a master in a school for young girls, and his life, passed in their midst, was greatly prolonged. "Accordingly," commented Hufeland (p. 6), "he gives the excellent advice to breathe the air of young girls night and morning, and gives his assurance that by so doing the vital forces will be strengthened and preserved, as adepts know well that the breath of young girls contains the vital principle in all its purity."

In the Eastern half of the world equal ingenuity was exercised in the attempt to rejuvenate the body and renew the forces of man. The successors of Lao-Tsé searched for a beverage that would confer immortality and have recounted extraordinary matters concerning it.

The Emperor of China, Chi-Hoang-Ti (221—209 B.C.), displayed extreme friendliness to the Taoists, believing that these had the secret of long life and immortality. In his reign, Su-Chi, a Taoist magician, persuaded him that eastwards of China there lay fortunate islands inhabited by genii whose pleasure it was to give their guests to drink of a beverage conferring immortality. Chi-Hoang-Ti was so delighted with the news that he equipped an expedition to discover the islands.[2]

[1] *L'Art de prolonger la vie humaine* (French translation), Lausanne, 1809, p. 5.
[2] A. Réville, *Histoire des religions*, vol. iii, Paris, 1889, p. 428.

Later on, in the dynasty of the Tchengs (618—907), when Taoism had again become a religion in favour at court, efforts were made to obtain imperial patronage for the draught of immortality, and magicians were in high favour. The Taoist writers called this drink *Tan* or *Kin-Tan*, the "golden elixir." According to Mayers, the chief ingredients of this marvellous compound were "cinnabar, the red sulphate of mercury, and a red salt of arsenic, potassium and mother-of-pearl. The preparation of it required nine months, and it passed through nine changes. One who had drunk of it was changed to a crane, and in this form could ascend to the dwellings of the genii, there to abide with them."[1]

The Taoists represent their saints, in the shade of willows, seeking the elixir of life, and in Chinese Buddhist temples there are placed votive cakes shaped like the tortoise, a sacred animal and the symbol of long life. Worshippers let stones of divination fall on these cakes and so ascertained if their lives were to be prolonged, promising for each subsequent year as many cakes as the divinity might demand.

The mysticism of the East reached Europe in the Middle Ages, and then, and even in modern times, drugs were used to prolong life. Cagliostro, the celebrated quack of the eighteenth century, boasted that he had discovered an elixir of life by the use of which he had survived for many thousand years.

There still exists, in some modern pharmacopœias, an "elixir ad longam vitam" compounded of aloes and other purgatives. Analogous preparations are known, such as the "vital essence of Augsburg" which is a mixture of purgatives and resins.

Serious physicians have rejected such preparations of the

[1] A. Réville, *loc. cit.*, p. 455.

quacks. They have abandoned the search for a specific, and, in their efforts to prolong human life, have relied on common rules of hygiene, such as cleanliness, exercise, fresh air, and general sobriety. In our own days, Brown-Séquard is an isolated instance of a seeker for a specific against senescence. This distinguished physiologist, setting out from the view that the weakness of old men is due partly to diminution of the secretions of the testes, hoped to find a remedy in the employment of subcutaneous injections of emulsions of the testes of animals (dogs and guinea-pigs). Brown-Séquard,[1] then aged 72 years, gave himself several such injections, and declared that he found himself reinforced and rejuvenated. Since then, numbers of persons have undergone the treatment which for a time was in vogue. The observations of physicians, made on old men and sick persons, have not justified the hopes which were entertained of the mode of treatment. Fürbringer,[2] in particular, working in Germany, has discredited the injections of Brown-Séquard. However, instead of following exactly the original prescription, Fürbringer employed a testicular emulsion which had been previously raised to the boiling-point. Brown-Séquard's method has not resisted scientific investigation, and although it is still occasionally employed in France, it has been given up in many countries.

Brown-Séquard laid stress on the efficacy of emulsions of testis as opposed to chemical substances prepared from the gland. Other scientific men, on the other hand, have attached value to such substances and in particular to an organic alkali the salt of which is known as spermine. That salt, made by Poehl of St. Petersburg, has been largely used. Several observers declare that its employ-

[1] *Comptes rendus de la Société de Biologie*, 1899, p. 415.
[2] *Deutsche medicin. Wochenschrift*, 1891, p. 1027.

ment, injected in solution or even absorbed directly as a powder, has been followed by a strengthening of bodily power enfeebled by age or labour.

As I have no personal experience of spermine, I shall quote from Professor Poehl[1] some indications of its efficacy. Several physicians (Drs. Maximovitch, Bukojemsky, Krieger and Postoeff) have given injections of spermine to enfeebled old men who had lost appetite and sleep, and have noted improvement lasting for months. From the instances given, I have selected that of an old lady of ninety-five years, afflicted with severe sclerosis of the arteries, with no appetite, a bad digestion and constipation. This patient had complained for several years of sacral pains, and moreover was nearly quite deaf and suffered from periodic attacks of malarial fever. The injections of spermine, given for a period of fifteen months, restored the old lady to such an extent that she recovered her power of hearing and felt the sacral pains only slightly and after a long walk. Her general condition was highly satisfactory.

Spermine, as it has been used medically, is prepared not only from the testes of animals but from the prostate gland, ovary, pancreas, thyroid gland and spleen. The substance is not specially associated with spermatozoa but has a wide distribution in the mammalian body.

In the medical treatment of the evils of old age, testicular emulsions or spermine have not been so favoured as general hygienic measures. Dr. Weber,[2] a London medical man, has recently summarised more general measures, and his evidence is the more important as he has been able to test

---

[1] *Die physiologisch-chemisch. Grundlagen d. Spermintheorie*, Berlin, 1898.

[2] *British Medical Journal*, 1904 ; *Deutsche Mediz. Wochenschr.*, 1904, Nos. 18-21.

SUGGESTIONS FOR PROLONGING LIFE 141

the efficacy of his precepts in his own case. Dr. Weber is 83 years old, and in his practice has cared for many other old men.

The following are the precepts which Dr. Weber formulated: All the organs must be preserved in a condition of vigour. It is necessary to recognise and subdue any morbid tendencies whether these be hereditary or have been acquired during life. It is necessary to be moderate in food and drink, and in all other physical pleasures. The air should be pure in the dwelling and in the vicinity. It is necessary to take exercise daily, whatever be the weather. In many cases the respiratory movements must be specially exercised, and exercise on level ground and up-hill should be taken. The persons should go to bed early and rise early, and not sleep for more than six or seven hours. A bath should be taken daily and the skin should be well rubbed, the water used being hot or cold, according to taste. Sometimes it is advantageous to use hot and cold water. Regular work and mental occupation are indispensable. It is useful to stimulate the enjoyment of life so that the mind may be tranquil and full of hope. On the other hand, the passions must be controlled and the nervous sensations of grief avoided. Finally, there must be a resolute intention to preserve the health, to avoid alcohol and other stimulants as well as narcotics and soothing drugs.

By following his own precepts, Dr. Weber has enjoyed a vigorous and happy old age. A Mde. Nausenne, who died on March 12th, 1756, at the age of 125 years, in the Dinay Infirmary (Côtes-du-Nord) explained the secret of her still greater longevity as follows: " Extreme sobriety, no worry, body and mind quite calm" (Chemin, *op. cit.*, p. 101).

Hygienic measures have been the most successful in prolonging life and in lessening the ills of old age.

Although until quite recently hygiene has rested upon a very small number of scientifically established facts, and although its precepts have not been followed rigidly, none the less it has already succeeded in increasing the duration of human life. This becomes evident if we compare the mortality tables of the present day with those of the past.

There is reason to state definitely that the mortality in civilised countries has decreased on the whole in the last one or two centuries. I have taken some facts regarding this from the valuable monograph of M. Westergaard.[1] That author came to the conclusion that the mortality rate in the 19th century in civilised countries was "much lower than in most earlier centuries." This diminution has been chiefly in infantile mortality. According to Mallet, the mortality rate of infants in the first year of their life was, in Geneva, 26 per cent. in the 16th century, and fell gradually to $16\frac{1}{2}$ per cent. at the beginning of the 19th century. A similar change has been reported from Berlin, Holland, Denmark and other places. However, it is not only very young infants that have shown a diminution in the death-rate. The life of old people has been prolonged to an extent equally remarkable. The following are some of the facts which support this statement. Whilst the old Protestant clergymen of Denmark at ages varying from $74\frac{1}{2}$ to $89\frac{1}{2}$ years had a mortality rate of 22 per cent. in the second half of the 18th century, the rate had sunk to 16.4 per cent. by the middle of the 19th century. This is not an isolated fact. The old clergymen of England (65 to 95 years) have also come to live longer, because in the 18th century the mortality rate was 11.5 per cent. and in the 19th century (1800-1860) only 10.8 per cent. There has been a similar decrease in the mortality

[1] *Die Lehre von d. Mortalitaet u. Morbilitaet*, 2nd edition, Jena, 1901.

SUGGESTIONS FOR PROLONGING LIFE 143

rate in the members of both sexes of the Royal Houses of Europe (Westergaard, p. 284).

From 1841 to 1850, in England and Wales 162·81 individuals out of every thousand of both sexes died annually, but the corresponding figure for the period 1881 to 1890 was decreased to 153·67 per thousand.

Westergaard (p. 296) has displayed in a most useful table the mortality in the chief countries of Europe and in the State of Massachusetts, in two periods of time. In the case of old persons from 70 to 75 years, there has been a constant decrease in the death-rate, without any exceptions. The exact statistics collected by Pension Bureaus and Life Assurance Companies exhibit the same general tendency.

It cannot be disputed then that there has been a general increase in the duration of life, and that old people live longer at the present time than in former ages. This fact, however, cannot be taken absolutely, and it is still possible that in particular cases there may have been more centenarians hitherto than at present.

The prolongation of life which has come to pass in recent centuries must certainly be attributed to the advance of hygiene. The general measures for the preservation of health, although they were not specially directed to old people, have had an effect of increasing their longevity. As in the 18th century and for the greater part of the 19th, the science of hygiene was in a very rudimentary condition, we may well believe that improvement in cleanliness and in the general conditions have contributed largely to the prolongation of life. It is now a long time since Liebig said that the amount of soap used could be taken as a measure of the degree of civilisation of a people. As a matter of fact, cleanliness of the body brought about in the most simple way, by washing with soap, has had a most important effect in lessening disease and mortality from disease. In this connection, the fact recently published by Prof. Czerny,[1] a well-known German surgeon, has a special interest. Although cancer, the special scourge of old age, has increased in recent times, one form of the disease, cancer of the skin, has diminished notably. " Cancers of the skin," Prof. Czerny says, " are met with almost exclusively on uncovered regions of the body, or on parts accessible to the hands. They develop especially where the susceptibility is increased by ulcers or scars which are easily soiled. And so it happens that in the classes where care is taken as to cleanliness cancer of the skin is very rare and certainly much more rare than it used to be."

M. Westergaard thinks that vaccination against small-pox has been of considerable importance in lowering the death-rate in the 19th century. This, however, can have had little effect on the duration of life in old people, as deaths due to small-pox in the old are excessively rare. For instance, in the second half of the 18th century, that is to say before the introduction of Jenner's method, the mortality from small-pox at Berlin was 9·8 per cent. of all the deaths, but of these only 0·6 per cent. were cases of persons more than fifteen years old. The rest, that is to say, 99·3 per cent. fell on children under that age. It may be supposed that most of the old people at that time were already protected by previous attacks of small-pox, contracted when they were young.

If hygiene were able to prolong life when it was little developed, as was the case until recently, we may well believe that, with our greater knowledge of to-day, a much better result will be obtained.

[1] *Medizinische Klinik*, 1905, No. 22.

III

DISEASES THAT SHORTEN LIFE

> Measures against infectious diseases as aiding in the prolongation of life—Prevention of syphilis—Attempts to prepare serums which could strengthen the higher elements of the organism

ATTACKS of infectious diseases incurred during life frequently shorten its duration and it has been observed that most centenarians have enjoyed good health throughout their lives. Syphilis is the most important of these diseases. It is not really a cause of death itself, but it predisposes the organism to the attacks of other diseases, amongst the latter being some particularly fatal to old people, such as diseases of the heart and blood-vessels (angina pectoris and aneurism of the aorta) and some malignant tumours, especially cancer of the tongue and of the mouth. To lengthen human life, it is a fundamental necessity to avoid infection by syphilis. To reach this result everything must be done to spread medical knowledge about such diseases. It is absolutely necessary to overcome the deeply rooted prejudice in favour of concealing everything relating to sexual matters. Complete information should be widely spread as to the means of protecting humanity against this awful scourge. It has now been possible to apply experimental methods to the investigation of this disease, and science has obtained a series of results of the highest practical utility. Prof. Neisser of Breslau, one of the most distinguished of modern venereal physicians, has summed up the present state of knowledge of these matters in the following lines.[1] "It is our duty as medical men," he says, "to recommend strongly as a means of disinfection in all possible cases of contagion the calomel ointment which Metchnikoff and Roux have advised." It is to be hoped that future generations, by following this advice, will see an enormous diminution in the number of cases of syphilis.

Syphilis, however, although a very important factor, is not alone in shortening the life of man. A very large number of persons die prematurely although they have not contracted that disease. We do not know the duration of human life before the arrival of syphilis in Europe, but there is no reason to think that it was very different from what it is to-day. We must, therefore, try to prevent as many infectious diseases as possible, and recent advances in medicine have made this task much less difficult. Pneumonia, it is true, the most common infectious disease amongst the old, cannot yet be easily avoided. All the antipneumonic serums which have hitherto been prepared have turned out to have little efficacy; but there is no reason to give up the hope that this problem will yet be solved.

Diseases of the heart, which are common in extreme old age, are particularly difficult to avoid, because in most cases we do not know sufficiently well their primary causes. In so far as they depend upon intemperance or infectious diseases such as syphilis, they can be avoided by the employment of suitable measures.

As the higher elements of the body in old people become

[1] *Die experimentelle Syphilisforschung*, Berlin, 1906, p. 82.

weaker and are devoured by the macrophags, it seems probable that the destruction or deterioration of these voracious cells would tend to the prolongation of life. However, as the macrophags are indispensable in the struggle against the microbes of infectious diseases, and particularly of chronic disease, such as tuberculosis, it is necessary to preserve them. We must turn rather to the idea of a remedy which could strengthen the higher elements and make them a less ready prey to the macrophags.

In the " Nature of Man " (Chap. III.) in discussing the simian origin of mankind, I touched on the existence of animal serums that have the power of dissolving the blood corpuscles of other species of animals. There is now, in biological science, a new chapter upon such serums, which have been called cytotoxic serums because they are able to poison the cells of organs.

The blood and blood serum of some animals act as poisons when they are introduced into an organism. Eels and snakes, even non-poisonous snakes, are cases in point. A small quantity of the blood of a snake, an adder for instance, injected into a mammal (rabbit, guinea-pig, or mouse) soon brings about death. The blood of some mammals is poisonous to other mammals, although in a lesser degree than that of snakes. The dog is specially notable from the fact that its blood is poisonous to other mammals, whilst, on the other hand, the blood and blood serum of the sheep, goat, and horse have generally little effect on other animals and on man. It is for this reason that these animals, and particularly the horse, are used in the preparation of the serums employed in medicine.

Now, these harmless serums become poisonous when they have been taken from animals which have been first treated with the blood or the organs of other species of animals. For instance, the blood serum of a sheep which has been treated with the blood of a rabbit becomes poisonous because it has acquired the power of dissolving the red blood corpuscles of the rabbit. It is a poison in the case of the rabbit, but is harmless to most other animals. The injection of the rabbit's blood into the sheep has conferred on the sheep a new property which comes into operation only with regard to the red blood corpuscles of the rabbit. We have here to do with something analogous to what has been observed in the cases of serums used to arrest infectious disease. When the bacilli of diphtheria, or their products, have been injected into horses, there is produced an anti-diphtheric serum, capable of curing diphtheria, but powerless against tetanus or plague. After M. J. M. Bordet of the Pasteur Institute had made his discovery of serums that had acquired the power of dissolving the red blood corpuscles of other animals, the attempt was made to prepare similar serums directed against all the other elements of the body, such as white blood corpuscles, renal and nervous cells. In the course of these investigations it was proved to be necessary to employ a certain dose of the serum in order to obtain the poisonous result. If smaller quantities of the poisonous dose were used, the reverse effect was produced. Thus a serum, strong doses of which dissolved the red blood corpuscles and so made them less numerous in the blood, increased the number of these when given in very small doses.

M. Cantacuzène was the first to establish this fact in the case of the rabbit, whilst M. Besredka and I myself did it in the case of man.[1] Since then M. Bélonovsky of

[1] *Annales de l'Institut Pasteur*, 1900, pp. 369-413.

DISEASES THAT SHORTEN LIFE

Cronstadt has confirmed the result on anæmic patients, treating them with small quantities of serum. He has been able to produce in them an increase in the number of the red blood corpuscles, and in the quantity of the red colouring matter (hæmoglobin) in the blood. Later on M. André[1] devoted much attention to this matter at Lyons. He prepared a serum by injecting human blood into animals and made use of it in the case of several persons who suffered from anæmia from different causes. In the case of patients, the anæmic condition of which had hitherto remained stationary, Dr. André found a sudden increase in the number of red corpuscles after injecting small doses of the serum. M. Besredka, in the case of laboratory animals, increased the number of white corpuscles by injecting them with a small quantity of a serum, strong doses of which destroyed these cells.

These facts are only a special case of the general rule that small doses of poisons increase the activity of the elements that are killed by large doses. In order to increase the activity of the heart, medical men give successfully small doses of cardiac poisons such as digitalis. As a commercial process, the activity of yeasts is increased by submitting them to weak doses of substances (fluoride of sodium) which, given in larger quantities, would kill them.

My general conclusion from these facts is that it is logical to lay down the principle that the higher elements of our body could be strengthened by subjecting them to the action of small doses of the appropriate cytotoxic serums. There is, however, much difficulty in putting this into practice. It is quite easy to obtain human blood to inject into animals with the object of preparing a serum

[1] *Les sérums hemolytiques*, Lyon, 1903.

which can increase the number of red corpuscles. On the other hand, it is extremely difficult to get human bodies sufficiently fresh to use them for a practical purpose. According to law, *post mortem* examinations can be made only after an interval of time in course of which the tissues have changed; besides, the organs obtained in this way are frequently affected by injuries or diseases militating against their use. Even in Paris, with its three million inhabitants, it is extremely rare that there is a good opportunity for the preparation of human cytotoxic serums. In two or three years, during which Dr. Weinberg has collected the organs from human bodies fairly fresh, he has been unable to obtain sufficiently active serums.

The best results have been obtained from new-born infants which have been killed by some accident in the process of child-birth, as in them the organs are in a normal state. However, owing to the advance in the practice of obstetrics, such accidents, already infrequent, are becoming extremely rare. In such conditions we may have to wait long before getting a positive result, unless the future will find some method of obtaining the necessary materials for this difficult and interesting purpose.

As it is so difficult to prepare a remedy which can strengthen the weakened higher elements of the body, it may be easier to find a means of preventing the weakening which interferes so much with our desire to live long. As the products of microbes are the most active agents in deteriorating our tissues, we must look towards them for the solution of the problem.

IV

INTESTINAL PUTREFACTION SHORTENS LIFE

Uselessness of the large intestine in man—Case of a woman whose large intestine was inactive for six months—Another case where the greater part of the large intestine was completely shut off—Attempts to disinfect the contents of the large intestine—Prolonged mastication as a means of preventing intestinal putrefaction

THE general measures of hygiene directed against infectious diseases play a part in prolonging the lives of old people, but, in addition to the microbes which invade the body from outside, there is a rich source of harm in the microbes which inhabit the body. The most important of these belong to the intestinal flora, which is abundant and varied.

The intestinal microbes are most numerous in the large intestine. This organ, which is useful to mammals the food of which consists of rough bulky vegetable matter, and which require a large reservoir for the waste of the process of digestion, is certainly useless in the case of man.[1] In the "Nature of Man" I have dealt with this

[1] According to a recent publication of M. Ellenberger (*Archiv. f. Anatomie u. Physiologie, Physiologische Abtheilung*, 1906, p. 139), the cæca of the horse, pig and rabbit, play an active part in the digestion of vegetable matter, which is rich in cellulose. At the end of his treatise, Ellenberger insist that the vermiform appendix of the cæcum is not a rudimentary organ. The reason why the appendix can be

question at length, as it was an important example of what I regard as the disharmonies of the human constitution. A case upon which I have always laid great stress is that of a woman who lived for thirty-seven years, although her large intestine was atrophied and inactive, as this seems to be a remarkable proof of the uselessness of the organ in the human body. The small size or complete absence of the large intestine in many vertebrates confirms my conclusion. None the less, some of my critics think that my argument is incomplete. To strengthen it, I may call their attention to a medical observation which is as valuable as if it had been an experiment. It relates to a woman, sixty-two years old, a patient of Prof. Kocher at Berne. She had been suffering from a strangulated hernia associated with gangrene of part of the intestine, and had to be operated upon suddenly.

The gangrenous portion of the ileum having been removed, the healthy part was implanted in the skin so as to form an artificial aperture through which waste matter from the food passed to the exterior without traversing the large intestine. Although the patient was old and seriously ill, the operation, performed by M. Tavel, was quite successful. Six months later, in a new operation, the small intestine was rejoined to the large intestine so that the fæces were again able to pass to the exterior by the natural channel. In this case, then, the large intestine was thrown out of use for half a year, not only without injury to the general health, but with the result that the patient was com-

removed in the case of man without disturbance to the functions of the body, is that this work can be performed by the Peyer's patches of the intestine. The existence of the appendix is not necessary to the normal processes of the body, and is a real danger to health and sometimes to life. Comparative study of the cæca in birds shows that these organs are in process of degeneration.

pletely cured and gained in weight.   MM. Macfadyen, Nencki, and Mde. Sieber[1] studied the digestive processes in the small intestine and the nutritive metabolism, and determined that these were active and healthy, the absence of intestinal putrefaction, that evil of the constitution, being specially favourable.

In six months of non-action, the part played by an organ

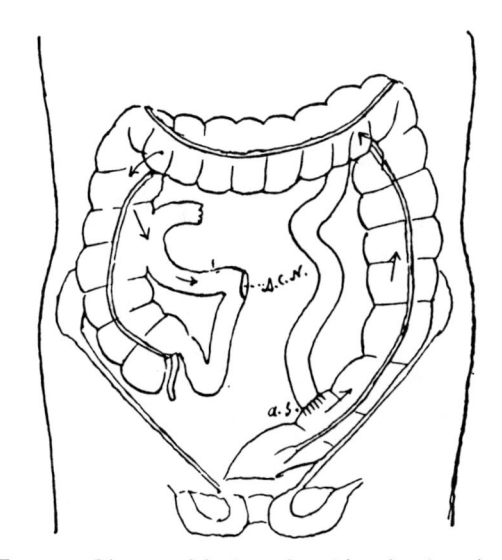

FIG. 19.—Diagram of the lower bowel in a female patient.
A.C.N., Artificial anus: *A.S.*, Insertion of the ileum to the colon.
(After M. Mauclaire.)

can be satisfactorily estimated. M. Mauclaire,[2] however, has put on record a case the history of which was longer. In 1902 he operated on a young woman and produced an artificial anus, there being no escape of fæcal matter by the ordinary channel. Ten months later M. Mauclaire operated a second time and shut off a portion of the intestine. He left the artificial anus, but cut across

[1] *Archiv. für experimentelle Pathologie*, vol. xxviii, p. 311.
[2] *Sixième Congrès de Chirurgie*, Paris, 1903, p. 86.

the lower end of the small intestine and inserted it near the iliac end of the descending colon (Fig. 19). For several days after the operation the fæces were passed by the normal aperture, as the small intestine now communicated directly with the large intestine, near the rectum. This condition, however, did not persist, for the fæcal matter began to flow back through the excluded portion of the large intestine, so reaching the artifi-

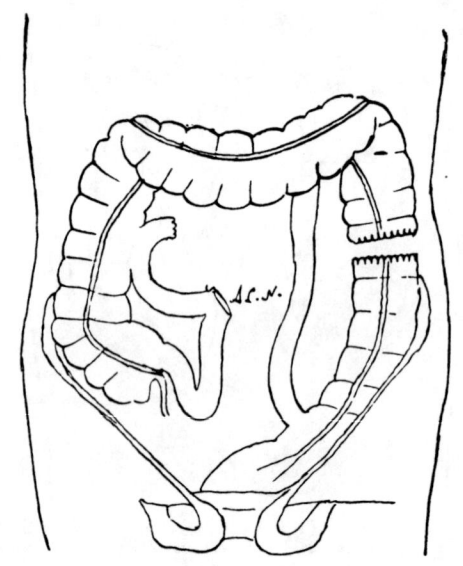

FIG. 20.—Diagram of the lower bowel, after a third operation, on the case in Fig. 19.
(After M. Mauclaire.)

cial anus, and causing inconvenience. Giving up the hope that this would cease, M. Mauclaire performed a third operation twenty months later. He cut across the large intestine near the point where the small intestine had been artificially led into it (Fig. 20), so dividing the digestive tube into two parts, one of which remained in communication with the natural anus, whilst the other, consisting of

PUTREFACTION SHORTENS LIFE 155

nearly the whole of the large intestine, communicated with the exterior by the artificial anus. In the new state of affairs, the food refuse passed directly into the terminal portion of the large intestine, and thence, by way of the rectum, to the exterior through the normal anus without being able to pass up the large intestine towards the artificial anus. In this last operation about a yard of the small intestine and the greater part of the large intestine, the cæcum, and ascending, transverse and descending colons were removed from activity.

By the kindness of M. Mauclaire, I have been able to watch his patient during the last four years. I satisfied myself that after the supposed exclusion of the large intestine, food dejecta ascended the colon and emerged by the artificial anus. There was such an accumulation of waste in the large intestine that fragments did not emerge until three weeks after the meal of which they had formed part. It was only after the final operation, that in which the large intestine was separated, that the dejecta escaped only by the natural anus, whilst a little mucus containing microbes was passed through the artificial aperture. Even three years after the operation, mucus continued to escape by the latter aperture, it being shown thus that after the large intestine had ceased to be a channel for the fæces, its walls continued to secrete although otherwise it had lost its function completely. Nevertheless the condition of this patient improved and she lived perfectly well without a functional large intestine. She takes food well but has to go to stool three or four times a day and has a tendency to diarrhœa. The excreta are smooth and often nearly liquid, especially after fruit has been eaten.

The case I have been describing, and which I am still keeping under observation, demonstrates once more the uselessness of the human large intestine; it should convert the most sceptical critic. But it also shows that the suppression of nearly the entire large intestine for several years does not completely get rid of the intestinal flora. Even without this evidence, however, I do not suggest that removal of the large intestine can be thought of as a means to prevent the pernicious effect of the intestinal flora.

Is it possible, without operative interference, to take direct action against the intestinal flora by the use of antiseptics? Consideration of this is already ancient history. When the theory that the intestine was a source of auto-intoxication was propounded, M. Bouchard[1] made the attempt to cure such cases by disinfecting the digestive tube with β-naphthol. He found, however, that that antiseptic, like many others, not only did not completely disinfect the intestine but sometimes had a harmful effect on the body.

M. Stern[2] has shown, in an elaborate memoir, that such antiseptics as calomel, salol, β-naphthol, naphthaline, and camphor, when administered in quantities compatible with health, do not disinfect the digestive tube at all. More recently M. Strasburger[3] has shown that when naphthaline has been given in quantities sufficient to impart its odour to the fæces, the intestinal microbes, so far from being diminished, are even increased in numbers. On the other hand, after meals consisting of milk to which there has been added an antiseptic in the proportion of a quarter of a gram to the litre, the intestinal microbes are really reduced in number. Strasburger obtained his best results with tanocol. Two persons who used, according to this method, three to six grams of tanacol per day, displayed a notable reduction in quantity of the intestinal flora.

Strasburger's conclusion was that "the attempt to destroy

[1] *Leçons sur les auto-intoxications*, Paris, 1886.
[2] *Zeitschrift für Hygiene*, 1892, vol. xii, p. 88.
[3] *Zeitschrift für klinische Medicin*, 1903, vol. xlviii, p. 491.

the intestinal microbes by the use of chemical agents has little chance of success." It cannot be denied that under special circumstances it is possible to decrease the number of microbes, especially in the small intestine. But this result is small and may be followed by the contrary effect, for the natural means of defence of the intestine against microbes are weakened, and the intestine itself may be harmed more than the microbes.

Strasburger, moreover, is no convinced advocate of the use of purgatives. The diminution of the sulpho-conjugate ethers in the urine, which certainly may follow the use of purgatives, does not necessarily indicate reduced putrefaction in the intestine, but may point only to a lessened absorption of the bacterial products. Such an interpretation is supported by an observed fact; in the case of a dog belonging to Strasburger, which had a fistula of the small intestine, the diarrhœa induced by calomel was accompanied by an indubitable increase in the total quantity of intestinal microbes.

Strasburger thinks that the most favourable results can be obtained by aiding the intestine in the discharge of its normal function. If it can be brought to digest the food more completely, there is the less pabulum left for the microbes. A similar result can be reached by lowering the amount of food taken, and to this course the beneficial effects of starvation in acute diseases of the intestine may be attributed.

The general conclusion, reached after many experiments on the disinfection of the intestine, is unfavourable. Very little is to be expected from the method. None the less I cannot regard the matter as definitely settled. Cohendy has investigated the effect on the intestinal flora of thymol which was administered in several cases with the object of destroying parasites. From nine to twelve grammes of thymol were administered to each patient in the space of three days, and there was a notable antiseptic effect, Cohendy believing that the quantity of microbes had been reduced to a thirteenth.

Such facts prove only that the antiseptic treatment is available up to a certain point. To attain the results, however, such large quantities must be used that the treatment can be applied only in special cases and at long intervals. More use can be made of simple purgatives which do not kill the microbes but eliminate them by the normal channel. It has been urged repeatedly that calomel, which is often used as a purgative, acts also as an intestinal antiseptic; but it is probable that its influence in reducing the intestinal flora is merely mechanical. It has been shown that calomel, like some other purgatives, lessens intestinal putrefaction, the evidence being the decrease in the sulpho-conjugate ethers in the urine. But although the diarrhœa induced by purgatives generally has such a result, spontaneous diarrhœas such as those of typhoid fever and of intestinal tuberculosis are associated with increased putrefaction.[1]

It is clear, however these matters may be settled, that regular activity of the bowels, increased by the occasional use of purgatives, must diminish the formation of intestinal poisons, and therefore also the damage done by these to the higher elements of the body.

When I asked the relatives of Mde. Robineau if they could tell me of any special circumstance which in their opinion had contributed to the extreme duration of the life

[1] There is a summary of this question in Gerhardt's work on intestinal putrefaction, in *Ergebnisse der Physiologie*, 3rd year, section 1, Wiesbaden, 1904, pp. 107-154.

of this old lady, they replied as follows:—" We are convinced that a slight bodily derangement, present for the last fifty years, has tended to prolong the life of the old lady. It cannot be said that she has suffered from diarrhœa, but she has been often subject to frequent calls of nature." It was most remarkable that the old lady showed no traces of sclerosis of the arteries. I may mention the strongly contrasting case of one of my old colleagues to whom a natural desire to empty the bowels came only once a week. A more frequent call was a sign of illness in his case. Now sclerosis of the arteries appeared in so marked a form that he died from it before he had reached the age of fifty years. This may be added to the list of facts which point to a close association between sclerosis of the arteries and the functions of the digestive tube.

Recently, at the suggestion of Mr. Fletcher,[1] the advantage of eating extremely slowly has been recognised, the object being to prepare for the utilisation of the food materials, and to prevent intestinal putrefaction. Certainly the habit of eating quickly favours the multiplication of microbes round about the lumps of food which have been swallowed without sufficient mastication. It is quite harmful, however, to chew the food too long, and to swallow it only after it has been kept in the mouth for a considerable time. Too complete a use of the food material causes want of tone in the intestinal wall, from which as much harm may come as from imperfect mastication. In America, where Fletcher's theory took its origin, there has already been described under the name of " Bradyfagy " a disease arising from the habit of eating too slowly. Dr. Einhorn,[2]

---

[1] *The A B C of our Nutrition*, New York, 1903; Dr. Regnault, Nov. 1, " L'art de manger," *La Revue*, 1906, p. 92.

[2] *Zeitschr. f. diatetische u. physikal. Therapie*, t. viii, 1904, 1905.

a well-known specialist in the diseases of the digestive system, has found that several cases of this disease were rapidly cured when the patients made up their minds to eat more quickly again. Comparative physiology supplies us with arguments against too prolonged mastication. Ruminants, which carry out to the fullest extent Mr. Fletcher's plan, are notable for extreme intestinal putrefaction and for the short duration of their lives. On the other hand, birds and reptiles, which have a very poor mechanism for breaking up food, enjoy much longer lives.

Prolonged mastication, then, cannot be recommended as a preventative of intestinal putrefaction any more than the surgical removal of the large intestine or the disinfection of the digestive tube. The field lies open for other means which may probably solve the problem more completely and more practically.

V

LACTIC ACID AS INHIBITING INTESTINAL PUTREFACTION

The development of the intestinal flora in man—Harmlessness of sterilised food—Means of preventing the putrefaction of food—Lactic fermentation and its anti-putrescent action—Experiments on man and mice—Longevity in races which use soured milk—Comparative study of different soured milks—Properties of the Bulgarian Bacillus—Means of preventing intestinal putrefaction with the help of microbes

AT birth the human intestine is full, but contains no microbes. Microbes very soon appear in it, because the meconium, the contents of the intestines of new-born children, composed of bile and cast-off intestinal mucus cells, is an excellent culture medium for them. In the first hours after birth, microbes begin to reach the intestine. In the first day, before the child has taken any food whatever, there is to be found in the meconium a varied flora, composed of several species of microbes. Under the influence of the mother's milk this flora is reduced and comes to be composed almost entirely of a special microbe described by M. Tissier and called by him *Bacillus bifidus*.

The food, therefore, has an influence on the microbes of the intestine. If the child be fed with cow's milk, the flora is richer in species than in the case of a child suckled by its mother. Later on, also, the flora varies with the food, as has been proved by MM. Macfadyen, Nencki, and Mde.

Sieber in the case of a woman with an intestinal fistula. The dependence of the intestinal microbes on the food makes it possible to adopt measures to modify the flora in our bodies and to replace the harmful microbes by useful microbes. Unfortunately, our actual knowledge of the intestinal flora is still very imperfect because of the impossibility of finding artificial media in which it could be grown. Notwithstanding this difficulty, however, a rational solution of the problem must be sought.

Man, even in the savage condition, prepares his food before eating it. He submits much of it to the action of fire, thus notably lessening the number of microbes. Microbes enter the digestive tube in vast numbers with raw food, and in order to lessen the number of species in the intestines, it is important to eat only cooked food and to drink only liquids that have been previously boiled. In that way, although we cannot destroy all the microbes in the food, because some of them can withstand the temperature of the boiling point of water, we can kill the great majority of them.

It has sometimes been supposed that cooked or completely sterilised food (that is to say food that has been subjected to a temperature of from 248°–284° Fahr.) is harmful to the organism and that much of it is not well digested. From this point of view protests have been made against the feeding of infants with sterilised milk or even with boiled milk. Although in certain cases sterilised milk is not well supported by infants, it cannot be doubted but that boiled milk and cooked food are generally successful. The large number of children brought up successfully on boiled cow's milk and the health of travellers in arctic regions are ample proof of this. I have been told by M. Charcot that in his voyage to the antarctic

LACTIC ACID AND PUTREFACTION

regions, he and his companions lived entirely on sterilised food, or on cooked food such as the flesh of seals and penguins. As they had no green food nor fresh fruit, the only raw food that they ate was a little cheese. Living under these conditions, all the members of the expedition enjoyed good health, and there was no case of digestive disturbance in the whole period of sixteen months.

It is obvious that abstaining from raw food, and so reducing largely the entrance of new microbes, by no means causes the disappearance of the intestinal flora already existing. We must reckon with that and with the evil that it does by weakening the higher cells of the tissues. As the part of the flora that does most damage consists of microbes which cause putrefaction of the contents of the intestine and harmful fermentations, particularly butyric fermentation, it is against these that our efforts must be directed.

Long before the science of bacteriology was in existence, men had turned their attention to methods of preventing putrefaction. Food, especially if it be kept in a warm place or in a moist atmosphere, soon begins to putrefy and to become unpleasant to the taste and dangerous to the health. Everyone has known cases of poisoning from putrid flesh or other food material. Foà,[1] the explorer of Central Africa, has related that once, when they were starving, he and his men came on the putrefying body of an elephant. The negroes rushed to lay hold of the carrion, but Foà tried to dissuade them, explaining that to eat flesh in such a state was as bad as taking poison. All did not listen to him, and three negroes, who had taken pieces of the body, swallowed them before they had been properly cooked. All three died in a few days,

[1] *Du Cap au lac Nyassa*, Paris, 1897, pp. 291-294.

with the neck and throat swollen, the tongue almost paralysed, and the abdomen inflated.

In another case, sausages made of putrid horse flesh caused an epidemic at Rohrsdorf, in Prussia, in 1885.[1] About forty people fell ill after having eaten the sausages, which, according to witnesses, were green in colour, smelt badly, and had a revolting appearance. One person died, whilst the others recovered after cholera-like symptoms. It is true that all putrefying food does not produce the same effect. MM. Tissier and Martelly[2] found no digestive trouble after having eaten food that was quite putrid. Everyone knows that the Chinese prepare a dish particularly pleasant to gourmets by allowing eggs to putrefy. Some decaying cheeses are harmful to the health, but others can be eaten with impunity. The reason of this is that whilst putrefying food may contain microbes and dangerous toxins, it does not contain them in all cases. On the other hand, we must take into account the different susceptibilities of people to the harmful action of microbes and their products. Some can swallow without any evil result a quantity of microbes which in the case of other individuals would produce a fatal attack of cholera. Everything depends upon the resistance offered to the microbes by the invaded organism.

Experiments on animals fed on putrefying food have also given varied results. Some animals eat it without any harm resulting, others have attacks of vomiting and show such a repugnance that it is impossible to continue the experiment.

Not only flesh and other animal substances, but vegetables can undergo putrefaction and fermentation (butyric)

[1] Gaffky and Paak, in *Arbeiten d. k. Gesundheitsamtes*, vol. vi, 1890.
[2] *Annales de l'Institut Pasteur*, 1903.

which make it dangerous to eat them. Many accidents have occurred in man as the result of deteriorated preserved fruit. Vegetables, preserved in silos to feed cattle, sometimes go wrong. "If, for instance, rainy days come after sunny days, so that the uncovered fodder is wetted again, the resulting ensilage is poor and has an extremely unpleasant butyric odour, so that the animals turn from it." Sometimes the fodder grows black in the silo, and acquires a special smell. "The animals will take it only in the absence of other food; their excreta become black, and if they are kept on such a diet for a time they waste in a marked manner."[1]

In popular practice, the value of acids for preserving animal and vegetable food and for preventing putrefaction has long been recognised. Meats of all kinds, fish and vegetables have been "marinated" with vinegar, as the acetic acid in that substance, the product of bacteria, wards off putrefaction. If the materials which it is desired to preserve give off acids themselves, the addition of vinegar may be unnecessary. For this reason some animal products such as milk, or vegetables rich in sugar become acid spontaneously and so can be preserved. Soured milk can be made into many kinds of cheese, and these last for longer or shorter times. Many vegetables can undergo a natural process of souring, when they "keep" without difficulty. Thus cabbage becomes "sauer-kraut" and beetroot and cucumbers pass into an acid state. In many countries, as for instance in Russia, the use of acidified vegetables is of great importance in the food-supply of the populace. Fresh fruit and vegetables cannot be obtained in the long winters, during which the people con-

[1] Cormouls-Houlès, *Vingt-sept années d'agriculture pratique*, Paris, 1899, pp. 57-58.

sume large quantities of cucumbers, melons, apples, and other fruits which have undergone an acid fermentation in which lactic acid is the chief product. During summer, milk, which acidifies readily, is the chief source of acid materials for consumption. The chief beverage is "kwass," of which black bread is the main ingredient, and this passes through not only an alcoholic fermentation, but an acidifying change in which lactic acid is the most important product.

Rye bread, the chief food of the populace, is also a product of fermentations amongst which the lactic acid fermentation is most important, but in other kinds of bread also there is a fermentation in which some of the sugar is transformed to lactic acid.

Soured milk, because of the lactic acid in it, can impede the putrefaction of meat. In certain countries, accordingly, meat is preserved in acid skimmed milk with the result that putrefaction is prevented. Lactic acid fermentation is equally important in the food supply of cattle. It is the chief agent that, in the process of preserving vegetation in silos, hinders putrefaction. Finally, the same fermentation serves in distilleries to preserve the must from which alcohol is prepared.

This short review is in itself enough to show the great importance of lactic fermentation as a means of stopping putrefaction and butyric fermentation, both of which hinder the preservation of organic substances and are capable of exciting disturbances in the organism.

As lactic fermentation serves so well to arrest putrefaction in general, why should it not be used for the same purpose within the digestive tube?

It is a matter of common knowledge that putrefaction and butyric fermentation are arrested in the presence of

LACTIC ACID AND PUTREFACTION

sugar. Whereas meat preserved without special care soon putrefies, milk in exactly the same conditions does not putrefy, but becomes sour, the reason being that meat is poor in sugar whereas milk contains a good deal of it. However, the scientific explanation of this fundamental fact is difficult. It has been shown conclusively that sugar itself cannot prevent putrefaction. Milk, for instance, however rich in sugar it may be, readily putrefies in certain conditions. Sugar preserves organic matter from putrefaction only because it can readily undergo lactic fermentation, and this fermentation is the work of the microbes described fifty years ago by Pasteur. That great discovery proved the part played by microbes in fermentation and founded bacteriology, a science equally rich in theory and in practice.

I need not pause to develop the theme that the antiputrescent action of the lactic fermentation depends on the production of lactic acid by microbes, because I have explained the matter at length in the tenth chapter of the "Nature of Man." If the lactic acid be neutralised, the organic matter soon putrefies, notwithstanding the presence of the lactic microbes. The most important point is as to whether lactic fermentation really arrests intestinal putrefaction. Several sets of observations have been made upon this matter. Dr. Herter,[1] of New York, injected directly into the small intestine of a number of dogs quantities of different microbes. To test the action of these on intestinal putrefaction, he investigated the sulphoconjugate ethers in the urine, as he believed, in accordance with current and well justified opinion, that these substances are the best proofs of the existence of putrefaction. He found that whilst the introduction of

[1] *British Medical Journal*, 1897, Dec. 25th, p. 1898.

quantities of *Bacillus coli* or *Bacillus proteus* increased the intestinal putrefaction, lactic bacilli notably lessened it. Herter found a notable diminution of sulpho-conjugate ethers in the urine of dogs which had been treated with the lactic microbes.

The experiments which Dr. M. Cohendy[1] performed upon himself during a period of nearly six months are still more interesting.

When Dr. Cohendy had proved that much intestinal putrefaction occurred during a period of 25 days, in which he lived on an ordinary mixed diet, he began to take pure cultures of lactic bacillus, taken from yahourth. In a period of 74 days, he took quantities varying from 280 to 350 grams of the culture.

Analysis of the urine during the progress of the experiment showed that intestinal putrefaction had notably decreased whilst the lactic bacilli were being taken, and that the diminution persisted seven weeks after the taking of the bacilli ceased. Dr. Cohendy gives it as the direct result of his experiment that the introduction of lactic ferment into the intestine definitely arrests putrefaction. He obtained this result on a diet consisting of 400 grams of soup, 150 of meat, 700 of grain-food, 400 of green vegetables, 300 of fruits and dessert and a litre of water. He came to the conclusion that the elimination of meat from the diet was unnecessary, as the particular kind of lactic ferment he employed was extremely active in inhibiting the proteolytic ferments.

Later experiments made by Dr. Cohendy showed that the lactic bacillus became so acclimatised in the human intestine that it was to be found there several weeks after it had been swallowed.

[1] *Comptes rendus de la Soc. de Biologie*, 1906, March 17th.

Dr. Pochon, assistant to Professor Combe[1] at Lausanne, has repeated on himself the experiments of Cohendy. He took for several weeks milk curdled with pure cultures of lactic acid microbes and obtained "results that were quite definite as to intestinal putrefaction." Analysis of his urine showed that there was a marked diminution of indol and phenol, substances which are certain indexes of intestinal putrefaction.

In addition to such observations on lactic bacilli there is a good deal of knowledge as to the effect of lactic acid taken in bulk. The result of the various observations[2] shows that the acid lessens intestinal putrefaction and lowers the quantity of sulpho-conjugate ethers in the urine. This fact explains why favourable results follow the use of lactic acid in many intestinal diseases such as infantile diarrhœa, tuberculous enteritis and even Asiatic cholera. The addition of this remedy to practical therapeutics is due chiefly to Professor Hayem. It is employed not only in the treatment of diseases of the digestive system (dyspepsia, enteritis and colitis), but is indicated also in diabetes and is used locally in tuberculous ulcerations of the larynx. As quantities up to twelve grams can be given by the mouth daily, it is plain that the system is tolerant of this acid. It is either oxidised in the tissues or excreted with the urine. In the case of a diabetic woman who had taken 80 grams of lactic acid in four days, Nencki and Sieber[3] found no traces of it

---

[1] Dr. Combe, *L'auto intoxication intestinale*, Paris, 1906. This valuable work contains much useful information on the subject.

[2] Grundzach, *Zeitschrift für klinische Medezin*, 1893, p. 70; Schmitz, *Zeitschrift für physiologische Chemie*, 1894, vol. xix, p. 401; Singer *Therapeutische Monatshefte*, 1901, p. 441.

[3] *Journal für praktische Chemie*, 1882, vol. xxvi, p. 43.

in the urine. On the other hand, Stadelmann[1] found a notable quantity of the acid in another diabetic patient who had been taking over four grams daily.

The general interpretation of the benefits gained from the use of lactic acid ferments is that they depend solely on the action of the lactic acid which they produce in preventing the multiplication of the microbes which cause putrefaction. Recent investigations made by Dr. Bélonowsky, at the Pasteur Institute, show that a lactic ferment isolated from yahourth and described as the Bulgarian bacillus owes its antiseptic powers not only to lactic acid but to another substance which it secretes. Dr. Bélonowsky has studied the effects of this bacillus upon mice, by adding to their previously sterilised food quantities of this lactic microbe. As control experiments he fed other mice on food to which lactic acid had been added in quantities corresponding to the quantity produced by the Bulgarian bacillus, or which had been mixed with other kinds of bacilli. Another set of mice were given normal food without the addition of either microbes or lactic acid.

Out of these groups of mice, those which had been given the Bulgarian bacillus thrived best and had most progeny. Their droppings showed fewest microbes, particularly microbes of putrefaction.

The next stage in Dr. Bélonowsky's experiments was to feed mice not with living quantities of the Bulgarian bacillus, but with cultures which had been sterilised by heat (120°–140° Fahr.). These mice lived as well as those to which living cultures had been supplied, and notably better than those supplied with pure lactic acid. It is evident therefore that there is some other product of this

[1] *Archiv. für experimentelle Pathologie*, 1883, vol. xvii, p. 442.

bacillus which favours life by preventing intestinal putrefaction.

Dr. Bélonowsky showed, moreover, that the Bulgarian bacillus cures a special intestinal disease known as mouse typhus.

The experiments which I have described show that intestinal putrefaction is to be combated not by lactic acid itself, but by the introduction into the organism of cultures of the lactic bacilli. The latter become acclimatised in the human digestive tube as they find there the sugary material required for their subsistence, and by producing disinfecting bodies benefit the organism which supports them.

From time immemorial human beings have absorbed quantities of lactic microbes by consuming in the uncooked condition substances such as soured milk, kephir, sauerkraut, or salted cucumbers which have undergone lactic fermentation. By these means they have unknowingly lessened the evil consequences of intestinal putrefaction. In the Bible soured milk is frequently spoken of. When Abraham entertained the three angels he set before them soured milk and sweet milk and the calf which he had dressed (Genesis xviii. 8). In his fifth book, Moses enumerates amongst the food which Jehovah had given his people to eat "Soured milk of kine and goat's milk, with fat of lambs and rams of the breed of Bashan, and goats with the fat of kidneys" (Deut. xxxii. 14).[1]

A food known as "Leben raib," which is a soured milk, prepared from the milk of buffaloes, kine or goats, has

---

[1] In the English authorised version as in the translation of Osterwald the word "butter" is used in place of "soured milk." Professor Metchnikoff follows the translation given by Ebstein in his work on the Medicine of the Old Testament.

been used in Egypt from the remotest antiquity. A similar preparation known as "yahourth" is familiar to the populations of the Balkan Peninsula. The natives of Algiers make a kind of "leben" not identical with the Egyptian form.

Soured milk is consumed in great quantities in Russia in two forms, "prostokwacha," which is raw milk spontaneously coagulated and soured, and "varenetz," which is boiled milk soured with a yeast.

The chief food of many natives of tropical Africa consists of soured milk. The staple diet of the Mpeseni is "a curdled milk, almost solidified." "Meat is eaten only on ceremonial occasions." According to Foà, a tribe of the Nyassa-Tanganyika plateau, like the Zulus, take milk only in the form of a raw cheese mixed with salt and pepper.

Dr. Lima of Mossamedes, in West Africa, has told me that the natives of many regions south of Angola live almost entirely on milk. They employ the cream as an ointment for the skin, whilst the milk, soured and curdled, is their staple food. M. Nogueira reported the same circumstances nearly fifty years ago after his journey in the province of Angola.

Just as cheeses vary in different countries, so curdled milk varies slightly according to the nature of the flora of microbes. Taking all the soured milks that are produced by natural processes, it may be said that the greater number of them contain not only microbes that produce lactic acid, but also yeasts that cause alcoholic fermentations. Kephir, which is prepared from the milk of kine, and koumiss, which is a product of mares' milk, are notably alcoholic. Koumiss is the well-known national beverage of the Kirghises, Tartars and Kulmucks, nomads

LACTIC ACID AND PUTREFACTION

of Asiatic Russia who are famous horse breeders, kephir is the native drink of the mountaineers of the Caucasus, the Ossetes, and some other tribes.

It has been supposed that the chief merit of kephir was that it was more easy to digest than milk, as some of its casein is dissolved in the process of fermentation. Kephir, in fact, was supposed to be partly digested milk. This view has not been confirmed. Professor Hayem thinks that the good effects of kephir are due to the presence of lactic acid which replaces the acid of the stomach and has an antiseptic effect. The experiments of M. Rovighi, which I spoke of in *The Nature of Man,* have confirmed the latter fact, which now may be taken as certain. The action of kephir in preventing intestinal putrefaction depends on the lactic acid bacilli which it contains.

Kephir, although in some cases certainly beneficial, cannot be recommended for the prolonged use necessary if intestinal putrefaction is to be overcome. It is produced by combined lactic and alcoholic fermentations, and as it contains up to one per cent. of alcohol, its use as a food for years would involve the absorption of considerable quantities of alcohol. The yeasts which produce it can be acclimatised in the human digestive tract, in which, however, they are harmful, as they are favourable to the germs of infectious diseases such as the bacillus of typhoid fever, and the vibrio of Asiatic cholera.

Kephir has also the disadvantage that its flora varies considerably and is not well known. There has been little success in producing it by pure cultures as would be necessary were it to be brought into general use. When it is prepared from a dried remnant there is the risk of stray microbes being included, and these may bring about pernicious fermentations. Professor Hayem prohibits its use in the case of persons in whom food is retained for long in the stomach. "When it is retained in the stomach, kephir goes on fermenting, and there are developed in the contents butyric and acetic acids which aggravate the digestive disturbances."[1]

As it is the lactic and not the alcoholic fermentation on which the valuable properties of kephir depend, it is correct to replace it by soured milk that contains either no alcohol or merely the smallest traces of it.

The fact that so many races make soured milk and use it copiously is an excellent testimony to its usefulness. M. Nogueira has written to me to say how much he was astonished, on revisiting after a long period of absence the district of Mossamedes, to find the natives so well preserved and displaying so few traces of senility. Dr. Lima has stated that amongst the natives of the region south of Angola "many individuals of extraordinary longevity are to be found." Although they are thin and withered, these old people are very active and can make long journeys.

Mr. Wales, a lawyer at Binghampton, U.S.A., has been so good as to make me acquainted with some extremely interesting facts taken from a work by James Riley which is now a bibliographical rarity.[2] In the narrative of a shipwreck of the vessel on which he made a voyage in 1815, James Riley states that the wandering Arabs of the desert live almost wholly on the milk of camels, fresh or soured.

---

[1] *Presse médicale*, 1904, p. 619.

[2] "An authentic narrative of the loss of the American brig *Commerce* wrecked on the western coast of Africa in the month of August, 1815, with an account of the sufferings of the surviving officers and crew, who were enslaved by the wandering Arabs on the African desert or observations historical, geographical, etc." by James , S. Andrus and Son, 1854.

LACTIC ACID AND PUTREFACTION

On this diet they enjoy excellent health, display great vigour and reach advanced ages. Riley estimated that some of the old men must have lived for two to three hundred years. No doubt these figures are much too high, but it is probable that the Arabs Riley encountered lived really unusually long.

Mr. Wales has examined Riley's work critically, and is of the opinion that that author was a well-informed, sagacious and conscientious observer.

M. Grigoroff, a Bulgarian student at Geneva, has been surprised by the number of centenarians to be found in Bulgaria, a region in which yahourth, a soured milk, is the stable food. Some of the centenarians, described by M. Chemin in his memoir, lived chiefly on a milk diet. Marie Priou, for example, who died in the Haute-Garonne in 1838 at the age of 158 years, had lived for the last ten years of her life entirely on cheese and goat's milk (*op. cit.* p. 100). Ambroise Jantet, a labourer of Verdun, who died in 1751 at the age of 111 years, " ate nothing but unleavened bread and drank nothing but skimmed milk " (p. 133). Nicole Marc, who died aged 110 years, at the chateau of Colemberg (Pas-de-Calais), a hunch-back and cripple, " lived only on bread and milk-food. It was only towards the end of her life and after much persuasion that she took a little wine " (Chemin, p. 139).

I owe to the kindness of M. Simine, an engineer in the Caucasus, the following communication, taken from the newspaper *Tiflissky Listok*, Oct. 8th, 1904. " In the village of Sba, in the district of Gori, there is an old Ossete woman, Thense Abalva, whose age is supposed to be about 180 years (?). This woman is still quite capable and looks after her household duties and sews. Although she is bent, she walks firmly enough. Thense has never taken alcoholic liquors. She rises early in the morning, and her chief food is barley bread and butter milk, taken after the churning of the cream. Butter milk is a liquid containing very many lactic microbes.

Mrs. Jenny Read, an American, has written to me that her father, eighty-four years old, "owes his health to the curdled milk which he has taken for the last 40 years."

Curdled milk and the other products of milk to which I have referred are the work of the lactic microbes which produce lactic acid at the expense of milk sugar. As many different kinds of soured milk have been consumed on a vast scale and have proved to be useful, it might be supposed that any of them is suitable for regular consumption with the object of preventing intestinal putrefaction.

From the point of view of flavour I find that soured milk, prepared from raw milk, is much the more agreeable. However, when a food is to be selected for consumption during a long period of time, we must keep hygiene strictly in view. It is certain, therefore, that the Russian "prostokwacha," as well as any other soured raw milk, must be rejected. Raw milk contains a large assortment of microbes, and frequently some of these are harmful. The bacillus of bovine tuberculosis, as well as other pernicious microbes, may be found in it. According to the investigations of Heim [1] the vibrios of Asiatic cholera, when placed in raw milk, survive even when the milk has become quite soured. In similar conditions the bacillus of typhoid fever remains alive for 35 days and dies only after it has been kept for 48 days in completely soured milk.

[1] *Arbeiten a. d. k. Gesundheitsamte*, 1889, vol. v, pp. 297-304.

As raw milk nearly always contains traces of fæcal matter from the cow, it sometimes happens that pernicious microbes are introduced from that source, and remain alive notwithstanding the acid coagulation of the milk. The lactic microbes certainly prevent the multiplication of other microbes, as, for instance, those of putrefaction, but are incapable of destroying them. Moreover, raw milk often contains fungi (yeasts, torulas, and oïdia) the presence of which is favourable to the development of such pernicious microbes as the cholera vibrio and the bacillus of typhoid fever.

Prolonged consumption of raw milk increases the risk of introducing dangerous microbes into the organism, and this possibility drives me to recommend soured milk prepared after heating. Theoretically, it would be best to sterilise the milk completely so that all the contained microbes would be destroyed. This, however, requires heating the milk to a temperature of from 226° to 248° Fahr., by which it acquires an unpleasant flavour. On the other hand, the pasteurising of milk at a temperature of about 140° Fahr. is not sufficient to get rid entirely of the bacilli of tuberculosis and the spores of the butyric bacilli. We have, therefore, to fall back on a middle course, and be content with boiling the milk for several minutes. By so doing we certainly kill the tubercle bacilli and the spores of some of the butyric bacilli,[1] there being left only some butyric spores and the spores of *Bacillus subtilis*, to destroy which a much higher temperature is necessary.

As some kinds of soured milk, such as "varenetz," "yahourth," "leben," etc., are prepared from boiled milk,

[1] See Grasberger and Schattenfroh, *Archiv. für Hygiene*, 1902, vol. xlii, p. 246.

it might be supposed that they fulfil the conditions necessary for prolonged use. A closer examination, however, makes us reject them.

Boiled milk, to make it undergo the lactic fermentation properly, must have added to it a prepared ferment. What is necessary is not merely rennet, as was formerly supposed, but a number of organised ferments, that is to say, microbes. In the preparation of these soured milks, a leaven is employed, one of the names of which is " Maya," and which contains not only lactic microbes, but several others. MM. Rist and Khoury [1] have come to the conclusion that the Egyptian " leben " contained a flora composed of five species, three of which are bacteria and two yeasts. The bacteria produce lactic acid and the yeasts alcohol. Although the result is that " leben " is a nearly solid substance, whilst kephir is a liquid, the two are closely similar. In both cases we have to do with coincident lactic and alcoholic fermentations, and my remarks regarding kephir apply equally well to the Egyptian " leben."

Through the agency of Prof. Massol of Geneva, I have obtained a specimen of the Bulgarian " yahourth." Working with his pupil, M. Grigoroff, M. Massol [2] has isolated several microbes from this milk, amongst these being a very active lactic bacillus. The same soured milk has been studied in my laboratory by Drs. M. Cohendy [3] and Michelson. They found in it a very powerful lactic ferment, which has been named the Bulgarian bacillus. This was the microbe employed in the experiments of M. Bélonowsky, to which I have already referred. More recently, it has been carefully investigated from the chemical point of

[1] *Annales de l'Institut Pasteur*, 1902, p. 65.
[2] *Revue médicale de la Suisse romande*, 1905, p. 716.
[3] *Comptes rendus de la Soc. Biologique*, March 17th, 1906.

view by MM. G. Bertrand and Weisweiler[1] at the Pasteur Institute. It proved to be an extremely active producer of lactic acid, supplying 25 grammes per litre of milk. The other acids which this bacillus produces, such as succinic and acetic acids, are formed only in very small quantities (about 50 centigrams a litre). Formic acid is produced only in traces. On the other hand, the Bulgarian bacillus forms neither alcohol nor acetone, two frequent products of bacterial fermentation. The bacillus also differs from other lactic ferments inasmuch as it has no action on albuminoids (casein, etc.), nor on fats. All these qualities make the Bulgarian bacillus much the most useful of the microbes which can be acclimatised in the digestive tube for the purpose of arresting putrefactions and pernicious fermentations, such as the butyric fermentation.

As in all the known soured milks (yahourth, leben, prostokwacha, kephir, and koumiss) the lactic bacilli are associated with a rich flora in which pernicious microbes may be met (such as the red torula, a microbe which predisposes to cholera and typhoid fever, which I found in the leaven of yahourth, bought in Paris), it is necessary to work out a method by which good curdled milk can be produced with the aid of pure cultures of the lactic microbes.

It was the obvious course to begin with the Bulgarian bacillus, as that is known to be the best producer of lactic acid. It coagulates milk rapidly, giving it a strongly acid flavour, but it often also gives a disagreeable taste of tallow. It is true that after it has been kept for a long time in the laboratory in the form of pure cultures in sterilised milk, the bacillus loses to a large extent its power of saponifying fats, the taste of the curdled milk being then more agreeable. If necessary, therefore, soured milk prepared exclu-

[1] *Annales de l'Institut Pasteur*, 1906, p. 977.

sively with the Bulgarian bacillus can be used. In practice, however, it is useful to associate with it another lactic microbe, known as the paralactic bacillus, as the latter, although producing less lactic acid than the Bulgarian bacillus, does not break up the fats and gives the curdled milk a very pleasant flavour.

As it is undesirable to absorb too much fatty matter, it is necessary to prepare curdled milk for regular use from skimmed milk. After the milk has been boiled and rapidly cooled, pure cultures of the lactic microbes are sown in it, in sufficient quantities to prevent the germination of spores already in the milk and not destroyed in the process of boiling. The fermentation lasts a number of hours, varying according to the temperature, and finally produces a sour curdled milk, pleasant to the taste and active in preventing intestinal putrefaction. This milk, taken daily in quantities of from 300 to 500 cubic centimetres, controls the action of the intestine, and stimulates the kidneys favourably.[1] It can therefore be recommended in many cases of disorder of the digestive apparatus, of the kidneys, and in several skin diseases.

The Bulgarian bacillus taken from yahourth or from soured milk, prepared from pure cultures of lactic microbes, can live in warm temperatures, and, as has been shown by Dr. Cohendy, is able to take its place in the intestinal flora of man.

Soured milk, prepared according to the receipt which I have given, has been analysed by M. Fouard, an assistant at the Pasteur Institute. When it was ready to be taken, M. Fouard found in it about 10 grammes of lactic acid per litre. Moreover, a large proportion (nearly 38 per cent.) of the casein had been rendered soluble during the fer-

[1] Soured milk can be taken at any time of the day, with or in between meals.

mentation, which shows that its albuminous matter is prepared for digestion much as in kephir. Of the phosphate of lime (which is the chief mineral substance of milk) 68 per cent. was rendered soluble during the fermentation. These facts all confirm the utility of the soured milk prepared from pure cultures of lactic bacteria.

Those persons who, from some reason or other, cannot take milk, may swallow the bacilli in a pure culture without milk. However, as the microbes need sugar to produce lactic acid, it is necessary to take with them a certain quantity of sweet food (jam, sweet-meats, and especially beetroot).

The Bulgarian bacillus produces lactic acid not only from milk sugar, but also from many other sugars, for instance, cane sugar, maltose, levulose and especially glucose.

Cultures of the bacillus can be made not only in milk, but in vegetable broths, or broths of animal peptone to which sugar has been added. The cultures can be taken in a dry form (powders or tabloids), or in the liquid in which the bacilli had themselves been developed.

A reader who has little knowledge of such matters may be surprised by my recommendation to absorb large quantities of microbes, as the general belief is that microbes are all harmful. This belief, however, is erroneous. There are many useful microbes, amongst which the lactic bacilli have an honourable place. Moreover, the attempt has already been made to cure certain diseases by the administration of cultures of bacteria. M. Brudzinsky[1] has used cultures of lactic microbes in certain intestinal diseases of infants, whilst Dr. Tissier[2] has used them in similar affections of infants and adults.

[1] *Jahrbuch für Kinderheilkunde*, N. F. 12 *Ergænsungsheft*, 1900.
[2] *Annales de l'Institut Pasteur*, 1905, p. 295; *Tribune médicale*, Feb. 24th, 1906.

From the general point of view of this book, the course recommended consists of the absorption either of soured milk prepared by a group of lactic bacteria, or of pure cultures of the Bulgarian bacillus, but in each case taking at the same time a certain quantity of milk sugar or saccharose.

For more than eight years I took, as a regular part of my diet, soured milk at first prepared from boiled milk, inoculated with a lactic leaven. Since then, I have changed the method of preparation and have adopted finally the pure cultures which I have been describing. I am very well pleased with the result, and I think that my experiment has gone on long enough to justify my view. Several of my friends, some of whom suffered from maladies of the intestine or kidneys, have followed my example, and have been well satisfied. I think, therefore, that lactic bacteria can render a great service in the fight against intestinal putrefaction.

If it be true that our precocious and unhappy old age is due to poisoning of the tissues (the greater part of the poison coming from the large intestine inhabited by numberless microbes), it is clear that agents which arrest intestinal putrefaction must at the same time postpone and ameliorate old age. This theoretical view is confirmed by the collection of facts regarding races which live chiefly on soured milk, and amongst which great ages are common. However, in a question so important, the theory must be tested by direct observations. For this purpose the numerous infirmaries for old people should be taken advantage of, and systematic investigations should be made on the relation of intestinal microbes to precocious old age, and on the influence of diets which prevent intestinal putrefaction in prolonging life and maintaining the forces of the body. It can only be in the future, near or remote, that we shall obtain exact information upon what is one of the chief problems of humanity.

In the meantime, those who wish to preserve their intelligence as long as possible and to make their cycle of life as complete and as normal as is possible under present conditions, must depend on general sobriety and on habits conforming to the rules of rational hygiene.

PART V

PSYCHICAL RUDIMENTS IN MAN

I

RUDIMENTARY ORGANS IN MAN

Reply to critics who deny the simian origin of man—Actual existence of rudimentary organs—Reductions in the structure of the organs of sense in man—Atrophy of Jacobson's organ and of the Harderian gland in the human race

SEVERAL critics of *The Nature of Man* have protested against my theory of the simian origin of man. Some of these found my arguments unsatisfactory and unconvincing. Others have attacked generally my suggestion that some anthropoid had been suddenly transformed to a primitive human being.

It is true that so long as we have little palæontological evidence as to the actual descent of man, we cannot discuss the subject without the aid of hypotheses. I think, however, that recent additions to knowledge confirm the theory of the descent of man in a way that ought to influence the most resolute opponents. I have in mind chiefly the arguments supplied by the embryology of anthropoid apes, and by the investigation of their blood. None the less, there are still many authors who maintain their opposition. One of my critics, Dr. Jousset,[1] enumerates certain differences in the structure of the skeleton in man and apes, and concludes that these radically separate man from apes.

[1] *La nature humaine et la philosophie optimiste*, Paris, 1904.

No one has ever doubted that man was not identical in structure with the anthropoid apes, or that he differs from them in several characters of the skeleton and of many other organs. The differences, however, do not justify any radical separation of the two. The unusual length of arm, upon which my opponents throw so much weight, is in harmony with the mode of life of apes, as these climb on trees and walk on all four limbs. The difference between apes and Europeans in length of arm is certainly considerable, but is much less in the case of some lower races, such as the Veddahs. In the Akkas of Central Africa, the arms are so long that the hands nearly reach the knees. The fœtus of Europeans also shows an unusual length of arm, probably an ancestral feature. It is only after birth that the arms become relatively shorter.

All the other characters different in man and the apes, are equally secondary. On the other hand, just as apes differ amongst themselves, so also, the different races show differences often strongly marked. M. Michaelis,[1] in a comparative study of the muscular systems of monkeys, has made known many details of the musculature in the orang-outan and the chimpanzee, and it appears from his investigations that, although there are some differences between these two apes, they are both closely similar to man.

There are many variations in the muscular structure of man, and these find parallels in the muscles of apes. This is also the case with other abnormalities of structure, some of which resemble the condition in mammals much lower than apes. An example of this is the presence of additional pairs of nipples, arranged symmetrically on the sides of the chest and occasionally found in human beings. A similar abnormality has been found in some monkeys, and

[1] *Archiv. f. Anat. u. Physiol., Anatom. Abtheil*, 1903, p. 205.

the best explanation of such an occurrence is that monkeys, like man, are descended from mammals which possessed several pairs of mammary glands.

The large number of abnormalities and rudimentary organs which may be found in man affords important evidence in favour of the descent of man from lower animals. Some authors, however, have tried to dispute this view and even deny the existence of rudimentary organs. M. Brettes,[1] amongst my opponents, has brought together most facts upon this matter, with the object of proving that such organs fulfil some function indispensable to the body and bear witness to the existence of a general plan of organisation. My opponent, however, confines himself to general propositions, laying much stress on a law of "the subordination of organs" without proving that rudimentary organs have an actual function. In *The Nature of Man* I remarked on the uselessness of the wisdom teeth, which are not cut until long after childhood and which are useless in mastication. In many human beings these teeth never cut through the gum, and their absence is no disadvantage. This is a typical case of a rudimentary organ. To maintain the contrary it would be necessary to prove that the wisdom teeth fulfil an indispensable function and that their absence was in some way harmful to the organism. No one has been able to show this.

The mammary glands in males are another case of rudimentary organs. The function of these, of course, is well known in females, but it is only in the rarest cases that they are active in males.

The organs of sense supply many cases of rudimentary structures. Animals which live in caves, in the dark, do not discern objects by sight, and in these cases the eyes are

[1] *L'univers et la vie*, p. 592.

rudimentary. It is quite impossible to deny the existence of rudimentary organs. They are extremely important guides to us in our investigation of the past history of the human race. The comparative study of the organs which are rudimentary in man and more or less well developed in lower animals is of fundamental importance in the problem of our origin.

The higher apes, or anthropoids, display reduction in some parts of the organs of sense. The organ of smell, for instance, is much less developed in them than in many other animals. Man has inherited the imperfect condition of this organ, and his sense of smell is much less developed than that of mammals which are lower in the scale of life. Man, however, because of his intelligence, has been able to tame domestic animals, such as dogs, ferrets, and pigs, and to make use of their acute sense of smell for tracking game or obtaining edible plants. The imperfect condition of the sense of smell in man in other cases is well replaced by his mental powers. He no longer recognises the approach of an enemy by the sense of smell, in order that he may take flight, because he has better means of defence than those of animals. It is not surprising, therefore, that the olfactory apparatus of man is much reduced as compared with that of lower mammals. In apes and man the nasal region of the head is much smaller than in their mammalian ancestors, and in the deep-lying parts of the system there are corresponding differences. Most mammals, for instance, and the dog in particular, have four turbinal bones, the purpose of which is to increase the surface of the mucous membrane of the nose, whilst in man there are only three, one of which is rudimentary.

The olfactory apparatus in most mammals contains a well-developed portion known as the organ of Jacobson, the probable function of which is to appreciate the flavour of food in the mouth. In man, this organ is in a rudimentary condition and cannot fulfil its function, as it is devoid of its proper nerve. This remnant, now useless, gives us information as to the evolution of the organ of smell in man. In the human fœtus, Jacobson's organ is not only better developed than in adult man, but it is also provided with a stout nerve trunk, which disappears towards the end of embryonic life. The organ, however, cannot perform any olfactory function. The human fœtus, moreover, possesses five turbinals which later on become reduced to three, and of these only two develop completely.

The history of the evolution of the organ of smell, as it has been made out by comparative anatomy and embryology, links this apparatus in man with the corresponding organs of other mammals by means of these useless rudiments, which, however, are important evidence in scientific theory.

The auditory apparatus also has become reduced in man. Many animals, in the struggle for existence, require a very acute sense of hearing, more so than man or some of the most intelligent mammals. We have all seen how horses raise their ears to hear better when there is the slightest sound near them. Monkeys and man have lost this power, and man sometimes tries to supply the defect by artificial means. When a lecturer, for instance, is not speaking sufficiently loud some of the audience put their hands to their ears, making a kind of trumpet which serves to catch the sound. The human external ear is supplied with muscles, but in most cases these are too feeble to move it. In very rare cases persons can move their ears, the muscles inserted to the shell in most of us being mere rudiments of those that existed in our ancestors.

In the organ of sight, the little fold in the inner angle of the eye, known as the semilunar fold, is of special interest. This membrane is a useless vestige of a structure much better developed in lower mammals. In the dog it is present as a small third eyelid, supported by a special cartilage provided with a secreting gland, known as the Harderian gland. In birds, reptiles and frogs, the corresponding structures are much better developed. Everyone has seen the delicate membrane which, in the case of a bird, may shoot out from the inner angle of the eye and cover the whole of the exposed part of the eyeball (nictitating membrane). In these animals, the eye is protected by this third lid, which has its own muscles. As in the dog, this third eyelid of birds and lower vertebrates is generally provided with a large Harderian gland, which produces a liquid secretion like tears.

In most monkeys, this apparatus is much reduced. Many of them have still a small Harderian gland and a weak third eyelid. In man, as I have already said, there are only vestiges of these organs, the gland being almost atrophied and the third eyelid represented only by an insignificant crescentic fold. In the lower races the fold sometimes contains a small cartilage. Giacomini found it twelve times in sixteen negroes, whilst in 548 white people it was found only in three cases.

The interpretation of these facts is not doubtful. This little fold is the last vestige in use of an organ which was useful only in our remote ancestors.

The organs of reproduction in the human race also show a number of rudiments. There remain even traces of a hermaphrodite condition, a very low degree of organisation, going back to extremely remote ancestors. The evidence given by the very large number of abnormalities that are found in these organs makes it clear that, in the long period of the evolution of the human race, they have been subjected to a series of modifications. Thus, for instance, there is occasionally present in women a form of uterus resembling that of the lower mammals, or even the double uterus of marsupials.

The evolution of man has been dominated by the great development of the brain and of the intelligence, and man, accordingly, has lost many organs and functions which were of use in his more or less remote ancestors.

II

HUMAN TRAITS OF CHARACTER INHERITED FROM APES

The mental character of anthropoid apes—Their muscular strength—Their expression of fear—The awakening of latent instincts of man under the influence of fear

The facts of which I have given a résumé serve to show that evolution always leaves definite traces indicating its successive stages in the form of rudiments. It is probable, therefore, that the pre-human mental functions or psycho-physiological qualities, which have so long a history behind them, have also left more or less appreciable traces. These, however, must be more difficult to find than rudimentary organs which can be made visible by dissection.

If we turn first to the animals most nearly related to man, we find that the living anthropoid apes show in the clearest way their close relationship with the human race, and suggest that their kinship with our remoter ancestors must be even greater.

The anthropoid apes alive to-day are animals inhabiting chiefly virgin forests, and feeding on fruits and shoots, although they do not despise eggs or even little birds. To satisfy their wants, they climb with the greatest ease. Orang-outans and chimpanzees climb slowly and carefully, whilst gibbons show a greater agility and more perfect acrobatic power. They may be seen throwing themselves from branch to branch across spaces of forty feet with the greatest precision. They play at the top of very tall trees, hardly grasping the branches through which they pass, making leaps of from twelve to eighteen feet for hours together with little apparent exertion.

To give an idea of the dexterity and swiftness of gibbons, Martin took the case of a female which he observed in captivity. One time she hurled herself from a perch across a space at least twelve feet wide, against a window which one would have thought would have been immediately broken. To the great surprise of the spectators it was not broken. The gibbon seized with her hands the narrow board between the panes, and then in an instant twisted herself round and jumped back to the cage she had left, performing this manœuvre with great strength and the most marvellous precision.

The muscular force implied in the above narrative is possessed by all the anthropoid apes. Battel, an English sailor who gave the first description of the gorilla in the beginning of the 17th century, stated that the strength of that animal was so great that ten men could hardly master an adult specimen. The other anthropoids, although not so strong as the gorilla, nevertheless display surprising force.

Edouard, the young male chimpanzee which I used in my experiments on syphilis, struggled so much at the least touch that it took four men to master him. I had to give up allowing him to leave his cage because there was no way of getting him back to it. Even quite young chimpanzees, females not yet two years old, cannot be handled easily. Although they are very friendly, my specimens used to resist with all their strength when it was necessary to put them back in their cages for the night. Two men had much ado to shut them up.

CHARACTER INHERITED FROM APES

Notwithstanding this great muscular force, the anthropoid apes are cowardly. They have no idea of their strength, but fly from the approach of the slightest imagined danger. My young chimpanzees, although their teeth and muscles were already formidable weapons, showed the greatest fear when I put with them animals even so weak and harmless as guinea-pigs, pigeons and rabbits. Mice frightened them very much at first, and it took them a considerable time before they got over their fear of so insignificant an enemy. When living in a state of nature the anthropoid apes scarcely ever assume the offensive. "Though possessed of immense strength," wrote Huxley,[1] "it is rare for the Orang to attempt to defend itself, especially when attacked with fire-arms. On such occasions he endeavours to hide himself, or to escape along the topmost branches of the trees, breaking off and throwing down the boughs as he goes." Savage[2] wrote of chimpanzees that "they do not appear ever to act on the offensive, and seldom, if ever really, on the defensive." When a female was surprised on a tree with her young ones "her first impulse was to descend with great rapidity and make off into the thicket."[3]

The gorilla, the strongest and most ferocious of the apes, has sometimes been observed to take the offensive. Savage, quoted by Huxley, said that "they are exceedingly ferocious, and always offensive in their habits, never running from man, as does the chimpanzee. The females and young, at the first cry, quickly disappear. He (the male) then approaches the enemy in great fury, pouring out his horrid cries in quick succession."[4] Only males

---

[1] Huxley, *Man's Place in Nature*. Collected Essays, vol. vii, p. 54.
[2] *Ibid.*, p. 60. [3] *Ibid.*, p. 62. [4] *Ibid.*, p. 67.

take the offensive, nor can this be of frequent occurrence, as one of the most recent observers, Koppenfels,[1] states that "the gorilla never attacks man spontaneously; he tries to avoid him, and, as a rule, takes to flight as soon as he sees a man, uttering peculiar guttural cries."

Which of these characters are preserved in the human race? Man is naturally feebler and less of a gymnast than the great apes, but his disposition is cowardly. One of the earliest signs of mental activity in an infant is the fear of surrounding circumstances. The smallest change in its balance or its being put in a bath cause it to show signs of real terror. Later on, it is alarmed when it sees any kind of animal, exactly in the fashion of a young chimpanzee. The most harmless spider is enough to frighten it.

Although mental culture subdues fear to a large extent, fear reveals itself more or less strongly from time to time, and it is on such occasions that we may find in the human being psychological relics of his ancestors. An analysis of fear is of special interest.

The first result of the emotion of fear is flight. Consciousness of danger sets our limbs in motion, and our instinctive desire to escape displays itself even when flight is more dangerous than what we wish to avoid. At the first alarm of fire in a public building, people rush towards the exits and in so doing often perish from their wish to escape. Even in the extreme of terror, the desire of flight is one of the earliest impulses. Mosso, a well-known Italian physiologist, in a monograph on fear, relates that when a Calabrian brigand was sentenced to death "he uttered a sharp cry, heart-rending and terrible, looked around him as if he were eagerly seeking for something, and then stepped backwards as if to fly, and threw himself

[1] Ménégaux, *Les Mammmifères*, p. 24.

CHARACTER INHERITED FROM APES

against the wall of the court, writhing, with arms outstretched, scratching at the wall as if he were trying to break through it."

Although in such a case it was futile and often is harmful, the instinct of flight from danger is inherited from ancestors from a time when it served to save life. Attempts to escape are not the only signs of fear. There is often a trembling fit which would make flight impossible. In Mosso's case of the Calabrian brigand, "after his struggles, cries and contortions, he fell on the ground in a motionless heap, like a wet rag; he became pale and trembled more than I have seen any other person tremble; his muscles seemed changed into a soft and quivering jelly." This condition of trembling inertia is another legacy from animals. Quivering of the muscles often manifests itself in terrified animals. Darwin[1] wrote of it, "trembling is of no service, often of much disservice, and cannot at first have been acquired through the will, and then rendered habitual in association with any emotion." The phenomenon seemed to him obscure and difficult to explain, a view shared by Mosso. The trembling of the musculature of the body is a generalised and exaggerated form of the movements of the cutaneous muscles in the condition known popularly as "gooseskin." The latter, however, is a relic of an adaptation useful to some animals. The hedgehog rarely takes to flight at the approach of danger, but stands still, and using strongly developed muscles, rolls itself into a ball. In birds and many mammals, the muscles of the skin cause erection of the feathers or hairs. These movements often are performed during fright, and according to Darwin,

[1] Darwin, *Expression of the Emotions in Man and Animals*, 1873, p. 67.

serve not only to warm the skin, but sometimes to make the animal appear larger and more terrifying to enemies.

Fear and cold alike cause contraction of the superficial blood-vessels, and, in man, excite the contraction of the minute rudimentary muscles inserted to the roots of the hairs. "Goose-skin" is caused by the contraction of these muscles, the condition being a functional rudiment, no longer serving to warm the skin nor to make the body appear larger. In a few exceptional cases, "goose-skin" can be produced voluntarily. In the normal condition, the rudimentary cutaneous muscles of man are immobile, and it requires some special stimulation to set them in action.

Fear, which is occasionally able to excite the contraction of the involuntary muscles, also stimulates other muscles against the will. Under the influence of emotions that powerfully affect the nervous system, and particularly under that of fear, contractions of the bladder and intestines may be so violent that it is impossible to prevent the voiding of their contents. Accidents of this kind are not infrequent in the case of youthful candidates at examinations. Mosso relates of a friend, a volunteer in the war of 1866, that he was seized with terror during a battle and that the utmost efforts of his will failed to make his body endure the terrible spectacle.

The involuntary action of the bladder and intestines during fear is a legacy from animals. The phenomenon is common in dogs and monkeys. Chimpanzees, when laid hold of, discharge their urine and fæces. At Madeira I had an unusually cowardly *Cercopithecus* monkey which when at all alarmed discharged the contents of the rectum. Quite possibly such a mechanism was useful for the preservation of the individual. The emission of various kinds of excretions is of use in the struggle for existence. In

CHARACTER INHERITED FROM APES 197

that way the fox drives the badger from its earth and takes possession of it, whilst polecats and skunks defend themselves against more powerful carnivorous animals by discharging on them fœtid secretions.

Instinctive fear is therefore a very powerful stimulant, awakening functions which are rudimentary and almost completely extinct. Sometimes it sets in operation mechanisms which have long been paralysed. Pausanias gives an example of a dumb young man who recovered his speech when he was terrified by seeing a lion. Herodotus relates that the son of Crœsus, who was dumb, on seeing a Persian about to kill his father, cried out: "You must not kill Crœsus," and from that time onwards was able to talk. These ancient narratives have been confirmed by many modern observations. A woman, for instance, who had been dumb for several years, on seeing a fire, was terrified and cried out suddenly "Fire!" after which her speech was restored. Such are cases of the awakening of a function which has been arrested only for several years. But fear can bring into activity other mechanisms which have been inactive from time immemorial.

Many different kinds of animals can swim instinctively. This is true in the case of most birds and mammals. There are some species which show a repugnance to water, but none the less swim well enough if they are thrown into it. Cats shun water as much as possible, but, none the less, can swim quite easily. Historians relate that Hannibal had great difficulty in getting his elephants to cross the Rhone. Some females were ferried across first, upon which the other elephants threw themselves into the water to pursue them and swam across the river without any difficulty (Lenthéric, *Le Rhône*, 1892, p. 81).

The lower monkeys can swim without being taught, but

the anthropoid apes have lost this power, and man also is without it. M. Volz[1] states that the different species of gibbons which live in Sumatra are separated by rivers. Their inability to swim makes these a complete barrier. It is probable that the lower races, in this respect, are better endowed than we are. It is said that in the case of negroes, children run to the sea or to rivers almost as soon as they leave the cradle, and learn to swim almost as quickly as to walk.[2] In the case of white people, many find it very difficult to learn to swim, and it is at least certain that swimming is not instinctive as in the case of our animal ancestors. Christmann,[3] the author of a treatise on swimming, states that the reason of man is a worse guide than the infallible instinct of the animal. Fear is able to stifle reason and to allow the instinct to come into play. It is known that children or adults may be taught to swim by throwing them into the water. Under the influence of fear, the instinctive mechanism inherited from animals awakens, and man soon becomes a swimmer. There are some teachers of swimming who use this method successfully. I have myself known an individual who learnt the art in that way, and M. Troubat, librarian at the International Library, has informed me that one of his friends, a journalist who died at Noyon several years ago, bathed in the Seine one evening at Neuilly when he could not swim. Unexpectedly finding himself beyond his depth, a sudden movement of fear saved him. Since then, he said, he knew how to swim.

Just as there are cases in which terror provokes flight,

[1] *Biologisches Centralblatt*, 1904, p. 475.
[2] J. de Fontenelle, *Nouveau manuel complet des nageurs*, Paris, 1837, p. 2.
[3] *La natation et les bains*, Paris, 1887.

and others in which it causes an arrest of motion, so also fear may do a disservice to a swimmer. Those who employ fear as a means of teaching to swim, know that they must intervene if there is real danger. It is true, none the less, that up to a certain point fear can awaken functions which have been atrophied for numberless generations, and that we can learn from it something as to the evolution of the human race.

III

SOMNAMBULISM AND HYSTERIA AS MENTAL RELICS

Fear as the primary cause of hysteria—Natural somnambulism—Doubling of personality—Some examples of somnambulists—Analogy between somnambulism and the life of anthropoid apes—The psychology of crowds—Importance of the investigation of hysteria for the problem of the origin of man

THE study of fear is interesting in other respects than those with which I have been dealing. It is also a primary cause of the obscure and complicated phenomena of hysteria.

Thus, for instance, amongst twenty-two hysterical women observed by Georget[1] the primary causes were: terror, 13 cases; extreme grief, 7 cases; extreme annoyance, one case. A patient of M. Pitres, of Bordeaux, first exhibited hysteria after being extremely terrified. A man with a tame bear had come to the village. The patient went to see the performance and elbowed her way through the crowd until she got to the front row. The bear, whilst dancing, passed so close that its cold muzzle touched the cheek of the young girl. Marie—for that was the patient's name—was terrified. She ran quickly home, and almost on her arrival fell on her bed in an attack of convulsion and extreme delirium. Since then the attacks have been repeated many times, and the delirium associated with them always turns upon the terror caused by the bear touching her.

[1] Quoted by M. Pitres in *Leçons cliniques sur l'hystérie*, 1891, vol. i.

A hysterical woman at the Salpêtrière is haunted by terrifying dreams. She thinks someone is trying to murder her, or to cut her throat, or that she is falling into water, and she keeps crying for help.[1]

Some of the most curious phases of hysteria are the paradoxical and extraordinary cases of so-called natural somnambulism, in which the patients, whilst asleep, perform all sorts of acts of which they remember nothing in their waking hours. Cases of duplication of personality are also known, in which the patients live in two different states without, in one of these, having the slightest remembrance of what takes place in the other. One of the most curious observations was that of the somnambulist who became *enceinte* whilst in her second state. In her first, or normal condition, she was ignorant of the reason of her physical changes, although in the second state she knew about it quite well and spoke freely of it (Pitres, *op. cit.* II, 215).

In the state of natural somnambulism the patients generally reproduce the normal acts of their daily life which they have acquired the habit of performing unconsciously. Artisans devote themselves to their manual work, sempstresses begin to sew, maid servants brush shoes or clothes, lay the table and so forth. Educated persons devote themselves to intellectual work to which they are accustomed. Clergymen have been known to compose their sermons in the somnambulistic condition, and to read them over to correct mistakes in style or in spelling.

However, besides somnambulists who during slumber simply repeat the usual acts of their life, there are others who do special things to which they are unaccustomed.

[1] Bourneville et Regnard, *Iconographie photographique de la Salpêtrière*, 1879-1880, vol. iii, p. 50.

It is these cases which are most interesting from my point of view. I shall take one case which has been specially well reported. A hysterical patient, a girl of 24 years of age, was admitted as an in-patient to the hospital Laënnec. One Sunday, she got up about one o'clock in the morning. The night watchman, who was alarmed, went for the night doctor, who witnessed the following scene. "The patient went to the staircase leading to the nurses' quarters, then suddenly turned round and walked towards the washhouse. The door of that being closed, she then groped for a time and turned towards the women's dormitory in which she had formerly slept. She went up to the top of the house where this dormitory was, and when she got on the landing, opened a window leading to the roof, went out of the window, walked along the gutter, under the horrified eyes of the nurse who followed her and who did not dare to speak to her, went in again by another window and went down the stairs." "It was at this moment that I saw her," said the night doctor; "she was walking noiselessly, her gait was automatic, her arms hanging by her sides, a little bent, the head erect and fixed, her hair disordered, her eyes wide open; she seemed like some strange apparition."[1] This is obviously the case of a hysterical subject, who in a normal condition was not accustomed to climb upon roofs and walk along the gutters.

Another observation, reported by Charcot, related to a young man, seventeen years old, the son of a large manufacturer, and of good address. Tired out by working for his final examination, he had gone to bed early. Some time later he rose from the bed in his college dormitory,

[1] Stéphanie Feinkind, *Du somnambulisme dit naturel*, Paris, 1893, p. 55.

went out by a window, and without accident climbed on the roof and took a long and dangerous walk along the gutters. He was awakened before any accident occurred (Feinkind, p. 70).

A case observed by Dr. Mesnet and M. Mottet was still more interesting. A lady thirty years old and extremely hysterical got out of bed in the night, "dressed herself, completed her toilet without help, removed the furniture in her way without stumbling against it. She was indifferent and idle by day, but strenuous at night in performing the most varied acts. I have seen her walking about in her rooms, opening doors, going down to the garden, leaping on seats with the utmost agility, running about, in fact doing all these things much better than in her waking hours, in which she got about only slowly and with aid" (Feinkind, p. 84).

Horst has related an extraordinary incident which took place in the sixteenth century. "A soldier walked in his sleep to a window, and with the help of a rope climbed a high tower, secured a jackdaw's nest with its young birds, and regained his bed, where he remained asleep until the morning."[1] Unfortunately there are not sufficiently detailed facts regarding this incident, and for fully described cases we must return to modern times. Dr. Guinon has related one case in ample detail. A man thirty-four years of age, by occupation an interpreter, was taken into hospital for hysterical attacks. "One night soon after he came under the care of the physicians, this patient, towards one o'clock in the morning, suddenly arose from bed, threw open a window and jumped across the sill into the courtyard of the hospital. The attendants on duty ran after him, and saw him hurrying away, undressed and carrying a pillow

[1] *Dictionnaire des sciences médicales*, 1821, vol. lii, p. 119.

in his arms. He traversed a series of gardens and walks, with the topography of which he was unacquainted, climbed a ladder and got on the roof of the hydrotherapeutic establishment, up and down which he proceeded to run with the greatest agility. Sometimes he stopped in his flight and rocked the pillow he was carrying, kissing and soothing it as if it were a child. Then he retraced the route he had taken." On being questioned next morning, he had not the faintest remembrance of his nocturnal exploit. "A similar fit came on him five or six times" (Feinkind, p. 108).

The same patient, "after having turned over in bed several times, seized a pillow and held it to his breast. He then got out of bed, and, in his nightgown, ran through the dormitory to a door leading to the lavatories. He opened the door, readily but with violence, and entered one of the closets. Then, still holding the pillow against his chest with one arm, by a gymnastic feat both difficult and dangerous, yet which he performed with the utmost precision, using his feet and the free arm, he got hold of the edge of the frame of an open window, through which he swung himself to the sill, alighting on both feet, after which, preserving the pillow carefully from contact or shocks, he jumped to the ground (the infirmary ward was on the ground floor). He then ran quickly to the opposite corner of the courtyard, passing the whole length of the great building at full speed, holding the pillow carefully. By a path which led round the building, he reached a corner where there was a tower supporting a great water-tank. A kind of metallic ladder, placed almost vertically and with rounded steps, led up the side of the tower to a sort of observation-landing which at one point was adjacent to the edge of the roof of the bath-house.

"The patient set himself to climb this ladder without any

hesitation, holding on by his free hand and placing his naked feet on the rounded steps with extreme precision. When he reached the nearest point to the roof of the bathhouse he leapt upon that, and at a running pace climbed the zinc roof to the crest, looking round him from time to time to see if his imaginary pursuers were near. He ran along the crest which was so narrow that his feet had to be placed alternately on either side on the slopes of the steep-pitched roof, a performance so dangerous that none of the officials would follow him, and which none the less he performed with complete assurance and without a single slip.

" When he reached the middle of the building he sat down on the crest of the roof, leaning against a ventilating chimney. He then took the pillow which he had been carrying carefully, placed it on his knees with a corner against his shoulder, and began to rock it as if it were a child, crooning to it, stroking it with his hand or with his cheek that he pressed gently against the corner. From time to time his eyebrows contracted and his looks hardened, and he gazed around him as if he were being pursued or watched, then gave a growl of rage, and took to flight again, carrying the pillow on his dangerous path. All the time he kept speaking, but we could not hear what he said. He saw nothing that was not in his dream; he did not understand when his name was called aloud; but he could hear, for at the slightest sound near him he rushed off again as if his pursuers were upon him. This episode lasted about two hours, during which he had climbed over all the roofs in the vicinity, defying our pursuit of him " (Feinkind, pp. 106-112).

I could give other similar cases, but I think that I have shown sufficiently that man, when in the condition of natural somnambulism, exhibits qualities that he does not possess in the normal state, becoming strong, adroit, and a good gymnast, like his anthropoid ancestors. The close resemblance between the manœuvres of Martin's gibbon, which I described earlier in this chapter, and the dangerous exploits of some sleep walkers is most striking.

The impulses to climb on roofs and poles, to run along in rain gutters, to climb a tower to take a bird's nest, are characteristic examples of the instinctive actions of climbing animals, like the anthropoid apes. Dr. Barth [1] defines somnambulism as " a dream with exaltation of the memory and automatic action of the nervous centres, without voluntary and conscious control." "The striking exaltation of the memory is the dominating condition. The extreme exactness of the memory of places displayed by the somnambulist makes us understand how he performs his nocturnal wanderings, doing almost without the aid of his senses numberless deeds of which he would be practically incapable in a waking condition." However, as such a patient performs new acts which he has never accomplished before in his own individual life, we must suppose that the exaltation of memory includes extremely ancient facts, dating perhaps from the pre-human period. Man has inherited from his ancestors a number of mechanisms of the brain, the activity of which is inhibited by restraints which have been developed later. Just as man possesses mammary glands which under ordinary conditions cannot secrete milk, so also, in his brain, there are contained groups of cells which are inactive in the normal condition, but, also, just as in some exceptional cases man and the males of several species of mammals are able to give milk, so also in abnormal conditions the atrophied mechanisms of other nervous centres begin to act.

[1] *Du Sommeil non naturel*, Paris, 1886.

SOMNAMBULISM AND HYSTERIA

The secretion of milk by males is a return to an extremely ancient condition in which both sexes were able to nourish the young; so, also, the gymnastic feats and the extraordinary strength of somnambulists are a return to a normal condition much less remote from us than lactation in males.

It is curious to find that, in some cases, natural somnambulism is associated with power to move the shell of the ear. I know two brothers, who, when they were young, used to walk in their sleep in the most typical way. One of them, a chemist, used to climb on a high cupboard, or simply walk about in the room. The other brother, a sailor, in a fit of somnambulism, climbed to the top mast of a sailing ship. These brothers, who were somnambulists, had the cutaneous muscles extremely well developed and were able to move their ears voluntarily.

In this case the abnormality was hereditary in the family, and the two daughters of one of the brothers were also somnambulistic and had control over the muscles of the ears. Here, then, is a case of the simultaneous recurrence of two characters of our ancestors: mobility of the ear and agility in gymnastic feats. M. Barth characterises the somnambulist as "a living automaton in whom conscious will is for the time being destroyed." According to him, the somnambulist "acts at the suggestion of circumstances, and what seem most extraordinary in what he does are in reality instinctive reactions." This description agrees well with my view that in natural somnambulism the instincts of our pre-human ancestors are awakened, instincts which under normal conditions are latent and rudimentary.

Sometimes, under the stimulus of fear, the instinctive mechanism of swimming is awakened in man. It would be extremely interesting to know if a similar occurrence took place in somnambulists. I have been unable to find in literature any sufficient facts upon this subject. I can quote only one case, and that with all reserve, which was published in the article "Somnambulism" in the *Dictionnaire des Sciences Médicales*. "It is related that a somnambulist who took to swimming during one of his fits was called by his name several times, and became so frightened when he awoke that he was drowned." It would be extremely interesting to collect more numerous facts on the instincts shown by somnambulists.

I have given a good deal of attention to natural somnambulism with the idea that I should find in it traits recalling those of the life of anthropoid apes. I think that the extremely varied phenomena of hysteria could supply us with other facts, useful in investigating the psychophysiological history of man. Perhaps some of the facts of so-called "lucidity" which are well established could be explained as the awakening of special sensations atrophied in the human race, but present in animals. It is known that in vertebrate anatomy organs are found which have the structures of organs of sense, but which are absent or quite rudimentary in the human body. On the other hand, it is known that animals perceive some phenomena of the surrounding world, for the perception of which man has no organs of sense. Fish, for instance, appreciate gradations in the depth of water, birds and mammals have a sense of orientation and can anticipate changes in the weather more exactly than our meteorological science. When under the influence of hysteria, man may possibly be able to recover these senses of our remote ancestors, and to know things of which he is ignorant in the normal condition.

Hysteria is common to man and animals. Amongst the numerous chimpanzees which I have owned, several have shown signs of hysteria. Some, when they were in the slightest degree annoyed, lay on the ground, screaming terribly, and rolling about like children in a fit of passion. One young chimpanzee used to pull out its hair when it was in a fit of temper. The view that hysteria is a relapse to the condition of our animal ancestors is supported by the conception of hysterical phenomena, suggested by Dr. Babinsky.[1] This well-known neurologist thinks that "the phenomena of hysteria have two special characters, the one being that they can be reproduced by suggestion in some cases with the most complete fidelity, and the other that they can disappear under the sole influence of persuasion." M. Babinsky thinks that "the hysteric patient is neither unconscious nor completely conscious, but is in a state of special consciousness." In my opinion the latter condition corresponds to the state of mind of our more or less remote ancestors.

Occasionally a man, under some sudden impulse, falls into a condition of extreme violence, and, being unable to control himself, commits acts of which he repents immediately afterwards. It is the custom to say that at such times the brute has awakened in the man. This is more than a metaphor. Probably some nervous mechanism from a remote ancestor has come into action, at the call of some stimulation. As our anthropoid ancestors and primitive man lived in tribes, it is natural that when men are grouped together, certain savage instincts should awaken. In this connection it is interesting to study the psychology of crowds. When man is surrounded by a great many of his fellows, he becomes particularly responsive to suggestion. This condition is characterised as follows by M. G. Le Bon,[2] the author of a study on the

[1] *Conférence faite à la Société de l'Internat*, June 28th, 1906.
[2] *The Crowd: a Study of the Popular Mind.* English translation, London, 1896.

psychology of crowds: "The most careful observations seem to prove that an individual immerged for some length of time in a crowd in action soon finds himself—either in consequence of the magnetic influence given out by the crowd, or from some other cause of which we are ignorant—in a special state, which much resembles the state of fascination in which the hypnotised individual finds himself in the hands of the hypnotiser. The activity of the brain being paralysed in the case of the hypnotised subject, the latter becomes the slave of all the unconscious activities of his spinal cord, which the hypnotiser directs at will. The conscious personality has entirely vanished; will and discernment are lost. All feelings and thoughts are bent in the direction determined by the hypnotiser" (p. 11). Man, under the influence of the crowd, gets into a condition like that of a hysterical patient and displays a state of mind identical with that of our ancestors. "Moreover, by the mere fact that he forms part of an organised crowd, a man descends several rungs in the ladder of civilisation. Isolated, he may be a cultivated individual; in a crowd, he is a barbarian—that is, a creature acting by instinct" (p. 13).

It is quite natural to find relics of our prehistoric past in all kinds of hysterical phenomena. We could reach extremely interesting facts regarding the tribal and sexual life of apes, if we tried to compare with them the phenomena of human hysteria. The passionate gestures which are characteristic of some hysterical cases could probably be explained in this way quite simply, and the wild cries uttered by patients in acute hysteria would be similarly explicable.

I think that just as anatomists seek for points of comparison between man and animals, as palæontologists make excavations to discover the buried remains of creatures intermediate between man and apes, so also, psychologists and doctors should investigate the rudimentary psycho-physical functions with the object of building up the history of the evolution of our psychical life. It cannot be doubted that in this branch of science new arguments would be found to support the already well founded theory of the simian origin of the human race.

PART VI

SOME POINTS IN THE HISTORY OF SOCIAL ANIMALS

I

THE INDIVIDUAL AND THE RACE

Problem of the species in the human race—Loss of individuality in the associations of lower animals—Myxomycetes and Siphonophora—Individuality in Ascidians—Progress in the development of the individual living in a society

IN the following pages I shall try to reply to the criticism on *The Nature of Man* that in that book I only considered the individual without thinking of the interests of society or of the race. I have been reproached for having lost sight of the truth that in the general course of evolution the interests of the individual must yield to the higher interests of the community. It was asserted, in fact, that by advising orthobiosis, that is to say, the most complete cycle of human life, ending in extreme old age, I was suggesting something to the detriment of humanity as a whole.

This objection rests on a misunderstanding which it will be interesting to clear up. I think that the complete development of the individual not only would not injure the community but would be of great advantage to it. Moreover, we must not lose sight of the fact that the individual has rights which must not be ignored.

THE INDIVIDUAL AND THE RACE 213

In the attack on my theory many facts were brought forward which show that in the animal and vegetable kingdoms the individual is always sacrificed to the advantage of the race. There is no doubt as to this, and in the course of this book I have given exact facts bearing on it. I instanced plants such as the Agave and some Cryptogams which die as soon as they have reproduced; I have also spoken of the small female round worms (*Nematoda*) which are brutally torn in pieces and devoured by their progeny. It would be difficult to find better cases of the sacrifice of the individual to the species. The rule, however, does not apply to man, who, in this respect, stands in a special position.

Since the arrival of man, several species of animals have disappeared from the earth. Man has played a large part in the destruction of the Moa (*Aepyornis*) of Madagascar, the largest member of the class of birds. He destroyed the Dodo of the Island of Mauritius and Steller's sea cow (*Rhytina stelleri*), a harmless relative of the Manatee, from the shores of the Aleutian Archipelago. Man is about to cause the extinction of several species of harmful carnivorous animals, such as the wolf and the bear, and possibly it will not be long before automobiles have replaced the horse, which would then become extremely rare. However, although he has destroyed so many other species, man has taken good care of himself. The progress already made by civilisation has considerably reduced our mortality. Every year, a large number of young infants are kept alive by the aid of hygiene and medicine. The decrease of war and of assassination has also played a part in maintaining the race. The position which man has acquired in the world makes it more likely that what we have to fear is too great an increase of population, and although the theory of Malthus has not been verified in all its details, it is still true that man could multiply on the face of the earth too abundantly. It is already clear that almost in the proportion that humanity stops the effusion of its blood in war, it tends to limit the propagation of the race.

As the future of the species seems to be safe, it is natural to consider in the first place that of the individual. In this respect the facts of general biology are of special interest.

Man is not the only social animal on the earth. Long before his appearance other living beings existed in organised societies. The splendid colonies of Siphonophora float on the surface of the seas, whilst in the ocean depths there are societies of corals of extraordinary variability, whilst again, on land, many kinds of insects live in highly organised societies.

This social life has been developed without external assistance, and without any code to regulate the conduct of the individuals united for a common purpose.

It will be interesting to give a slight survey of the fundamental principles of such societies; I intend to draw special attention to one of the essential points in the societies of animals, hoping to elucidate the relations between the individuals and society.

In the organisation of human society the most difficult points are the extent to which the society may encroach on the individual and the degree to which the individual may preserve his rights and his independence. Disputes on these have been interminable, and I do not propose to discuss the theories according to which an individual must be sacrificed for the good of the community to which he belongs. I shall limit myself to reviewing the fate of the individuals in societies of beings much inferior to man.

THE INDIVIDUAL AND THE RACE 215

There are examples of societies composed of many individuals, even amongst living things on the borderland between the animal and vegetable kingdoms.

There may be found in woods, on dead leaves or on decaying timber, minute plants resembling tiny mushrooms. These are Myxomycetes, and the visible portions are minute sacs filled with microscopical rounded bodies, known as spores. When one of the spores is moistened, there emerges a minute organism with a mobile appendage

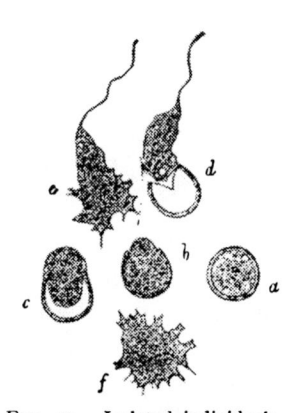

FIG. 21.—Isolated individuals of a Myxomycete.
(After Zopff.)
a, spore; b—f, escape of the zoospores.

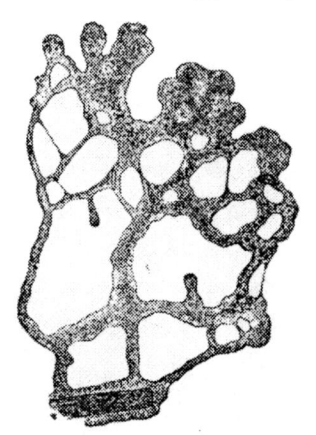

FIG. 22. — Myxomycete individuals united to form a plasmodium.
(After Zopff.)

by which it can be impelled through water. A drop of water on a leaf or on a fragment of timber may be filled with numbers of these tiny swimming bodies (Fig. 21). Their free life as individuals, however, is of brief duration. When they come into contact, their bodies fuse, forming a gelatinous mass which may be quite large (Fig. 22). This mass is called a plasmodium, and is composed of a living substance which can move slowly over leaves and which exhibits streaming movements in the interior, so that the whole resembles in some respects the lava from a volcano.

The plasmodia may be regarded as societies in the constitution of which the individuality of the members has been completely sacrificed. The ideal of those philosophers who have urged that man should renounce his individuality and merge himself in the community has been realised in the fullest way at the lower end of the scale of life, at an epoch inconceivably remote from the appearance of the human race.

Amongst animals, even the most lowly, there are no societies in which the members are sacrificed so completely to the whole. Individuality is always preserved to a greater or lesser extent. Consider the polyps, colonies of which form reefs in the sea and may even become islands. These creatures live in aggregations, the members of which are incapable of living an independent life. They are united by living substance and resemble double monsters, such as Doodica and Radica, who were so much talked of some years ago when M. Doyen operated upon them. The peritoneal cavities of these twins were in free communication, and the blood-vessels were united so that the blood of the one passed freely into the body of the other. In another double monster, the two Tscheck girls, Rosa and Josepha, the intestinal tracts communicate, both leading to a common rectum. In these, who are still alive, the peritoneum is joined and there is a single urethra.

In the case of the coral polyps, the fusion of the individuals of the colony is nearly always much more complete. Each individual has its own mouth and stomach, whilst the other organs cannot be assigned to individuals but must be regarded as common to the whole.

THE INDIVIDUAL AND THE RACE 217

In the swimming polyps or Siphonophora, the loss of individuality is still more remarkable. These graceful and transparent creatures, sometimes large in size, live in the sea and may appear on its surface in great numbers. They possess many whip-like filaments provided with tentacles, swimming bells and stomachs. There can be no doubt as to their colonial nature (Fig. 23), but it is difficult to decide as to whether each piece of the colony, each swimming bell, stomach and so forth, is to be regarded as an individual or an organ, different zoologists having taken different views on the question. One interpretation is that colonial life has brought with it such modifications that of each individual there remains only a single organ. Some individuals have been reduced to simple stomachs, attached to the central stem, whilst others have lost all organs except that of locomotion which has become one of the swimming bells of the colony. Other zoologists, and I myself amongst them, think that the Siphonophora are colonies of organs in which there has been as yet practically no development of individuality.

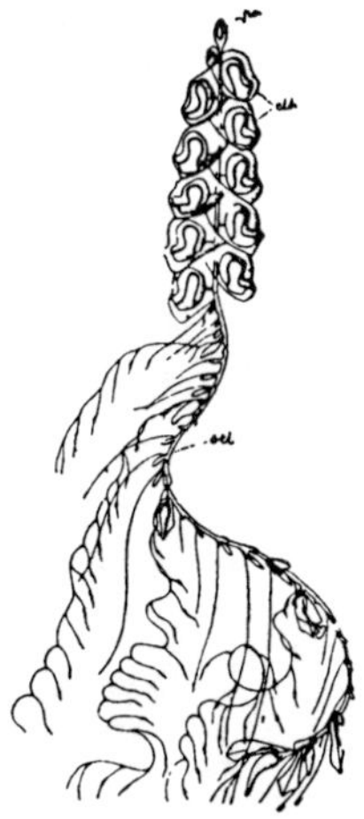

FIG. 23.—One of the Siphonophora. (After Chun.)
pn, pneumatic chamber; *clh*, swimming bells; *stl*, stolon.

A living chain of Siphonophora is simply a number of organs such as stomachs, tentacles, swimming bells and so forth, united on a common stem. I need not discuss the disputed point further, for the only matter pertinent to my argument is that in the Siphonophora the loss of individuality, the sacrifice of the parts to the whole, is not so great as in the Myxomycetes.

In support of my view, I must recall the small forms of Siphonophora known as *Eudoxia*. These are detached pieces of the common trunk which swim freely in the sea and have a remarkable structure (Fig. 24). Their mobility is due to a bell provided with strong muscular fibres. The bell is a portion of an individual which possesses organs of reproduction but which is devoid of the means to capture or digest food. These two functions are performed by a second individual which is closely united with the first. The nutrient individual has a long

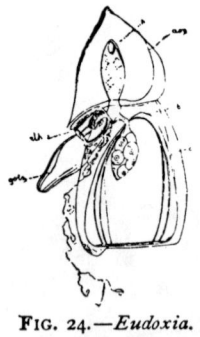

FIG. 24.—*Eudoxia*. (After Chun.)

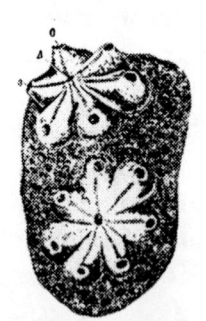

FIG. 25. — *Botryllus* colonies. *o*, mouth ; *A*, common cloaca.

tentacle by which the prey is captured, and a capacious stomach in which it is digested. The products of digestion pass by channels into the reproductive individual, carrying as it were a ready-made blood. *Eudoxia* in fact is a double being composed of an individual incapable of locomotion or of reproduction, but adapted for prehension and digestion, and of a second individual which can reproduce and which is mobile. *Eudoxia* is an association resembling that of the blind man and the paralytic, in Florian's fable.

Advance in the organisation of social animals is plainly

THE INDIVIDUAL AND THE RACE

incompatible with complete loss of individuality, and this becomes the more apparent the higher we reach in the scale of life. In the social Ascidians, each member retains all the organs necessary to life. Animals of the genus *Botryllus* (Fig. 25), perhaps the most interesting of these Ascidians, occur in the form of circular colonies. The individuals which compose the colony are grouped radially around a common centre which is occupied by the cloaca. Each individual has its own mouth and digestive tube, but the latter opens into a cloaca, common to all the individuals, by which the excreta are voided. There is, in fact, a single anus, as in the case of Rosa and Josepha which I have just mentioned.

II

INSECT SOCIETIES

Social life of insects—Development and preservation of individuality in colonies of insects—Division of labour and sacrifice of individuality in some insects

HITHERTO I have dealt with associations of animals the members of which are linked by an actual material bond. In the insect world there are many cases of highly developed colonies. But the organisation of insects is high, and is incompatible with the existence of actual physical connection between the members of the society.

In early stages of the development of the social instinct in bees, fully formed and similar individuals join together with the object of securing the safety of their individual lives. Sometimes they act together to drive away a common enemy, sometimes, as in winter, they cling in a mass to maintain their temperature. In such primitive societies, the young are not reared in common. It is only in much more highly developed colonies, such as those of some bees and wasps, and of ants and termites, that the chief object of the common action is care of the progeny. Such an extreme development of the colony is attained only by sacrificing the individuality of the members. There is a far-reaching division of labour, so that the queens, for instance, are mere machines for laying eggs. In hive-bees the queen can no longer judge of what is good for the colony, her intellectual functions being degenerate. She is enclosed in her cell and supported by the workers, who see in her the future of the race. In times of want the worker-bees sacrifice their own lives and give the queen the last remnants of the food-supply so that she survives them. The males are incomplete individuals and are tolerated only so long as they are required, after which the workers kill them remorselessly.

The workers, which take such pains for the well-being of the hive, are incomplete individuals. Their brains are well developed and they are well equipped with organs for making wax and collecting food, but their reproductive organs are reduced to mere vestiges incapable of fulfilling their functions.

Here then is a case of loss of individual characters increasing with the perfection of the colony. Amongst ants and termites, the social life of which arose quite independently of that of bees, the same course of events has been repeated. High intelligence and skill are confined to the workers, in which the reproductive organs are atrophied. The soldiers have powerful jaws used in defence of the camp, but they, too, are sexually incomplete. The females and males, in which the reproductive organs have attained huge proportions so that the bodies are little more than sacs containing the sexual elements, have no intelligence and very little skill.

An extremely curious specialisation, consisting in the formation of honey-bearing workers, occurs in some Mexican ants. Some of the workers of these races absorb so much honey that their bodies become swollen honey-bags. The limbs can no longer support the expanded body, and the insects, reduced to immobility, do not quit the burrows.

Normal life has become impossible for these individuals, who soon die for the good of the community. When the normal workers or the sexual individuals are hungry, they approach the honey-bearers and take honey from their mouths. The honey-bearers have become no more than animated cupboards (Fig. 26).

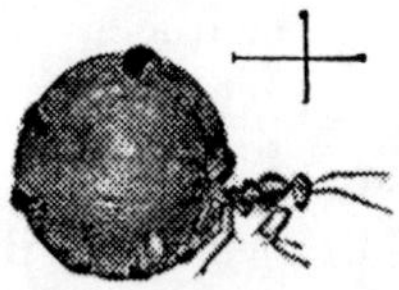

FIG. 26.—A Honey-ant. (After Brehm.)

The termites belong to quite another class of the group Insecta, but in their case a similar sacrifice of the individual to the state is practised. The females become transformed to shapeless bags of eggs. They cannot move, but remain secluded in the recesses of the "ant"-hill, where they lay as many as 80,000 eggs a day. The soldiers have become provided with jaws so enormous that these unsexed insects can perform no function other than defence of the colony.

The partial reduction of individuality in social insects never goes so far as in the cases of the lower animals I have described. It may be stated as a general rule that increase in the perfection of organisation brings with it a more or less complete preservation of individuality in the members of a community.

I shall now examine to what extent this law can be applied in the case of man.

III

SOCIETY AND THE INDIVIDUAL IN THE HUMAN RACE

Human societies—Differentiation in the human race—Learned women—Habits of a bee, *Halictus quadricinctus*—Collectivist theories—Criticisms by Herbert Spencer and Nietzsche—Progress of individuality in the societies of higher beings

Social life is for the most part little developed amongst vertebrate animals. The birds and fishes which live in communities present no organisation of society even comparable with that found amongst insects. There is little advance in this respect in the case of mammals, and it is not until we come to man that highly organised societies are to be found. Man is the first vertebrate to develop an organised social life. But, whilst in the insect world, instincts are of supreme importance in the regulation of the community, there is little instinctive action in human communities. The consciousness of individuality, or egoism, is very powerful in human beings, and perhaps for that reason our ancestors made little progress in the development of social relations.

Anthropoid apes adhere in little groups or in families without any true social organisation. Love of the neighbour, or altruism, appears to be a recent and feeble human acquisition.

Although the organisation of human society is far advanced and division of labour very complete, there is no differentiation of the individuals comparable with what is found amongst insects. Although in animals so different as Siphonophora, bees, wasps, and termites the development of the community, proceeding along different lines, has brought into existence non-sexual individuals, there is no trace of this specialisation amongst human beings.

Certain abnormalities in the condition of the sexual organs are occasionally found in men and women, but these cannot be compared with the production of sexless individuals that has taken place amongst other social creatures. I cannot accept the view that we are to see something analogous to the case of worker bees in the prohibition of sexual relations imposed by some religious systems on a certain number of individuals. But in any event there is little importance in this occurrence, which is rapidly becoming rarer.

In recent times, both in Europe and the United States of America, there has been an active development of a feminist movement impelling women towards higher education. Women, no longer content with the avocations of mother and housewife, have pressed into professions such as law and medicine. There is a steady increase in the number of women who study at the Universities, and countries like Germany, which have tried to exclude women from higher studies, will soon have to yield before an irresistible pressure.

Can we regard the results of this movement as analogous to the production of sexless workers which has taken place amongst social insects? I think not. It is undoubtedly true that a certain number of young women, who, for some reason or other are unlikely to marry, devote themselves to scientific study. In these cases, however, celibacy is the cause, not the result of the increased intellectual

SOCIETY AND THE INDIVIDUAL 225

activity. On the other hand, it must be remembered that many women students of science eventually marry. In St. Petersburg, for instance, there were 1,091 women in the Medical School; of these 80 were already married and 19 were widows. Of the remaining 992, 436 or 44 per cent. married during the course of their studies.

Observation of the femininist movement, which has lasted for more than forty years, shows that in most cases there is no tendency towards the formation of individuals resembling the infertile worker insects. Most lady doctors and learned women would like nothing better than to be the founders of a family. Even the women who have been most distinguished in the scientific world are no exception to the rule. In this relation it is very interesting to follow the details of the life of Sophie Kowalevsky, one of the most notable of learned women. In her youth, when she began to study mathematics, she would not admit that feelings of love had any importance. Later on, however, when she felt herself growing old, these sentiments awoke in her to such an extent that on the day when the prize of the Academy of Sciences was bestowed on her, she wrote to one of her friends, " I am getting innumerable letters of congratulation, but by the strange irony of fate, I have never felt so unhappy."

The cause of this discontent reveals itself in the words which she addressed to her most intimate woman friend. " Why is it," she said, " that no one loves me? I could give more than most women, and while the most ordinary women are loved, as for me, I am not loved."[1]

It is, in fact, impossible to regard the celibacy of persons devoted to religion or to scientific studies as the beginning of a special organisation analogous to that of worker bees.

[1] *Souvenirs d'enfance de S. Kowalevsky*, 1895, pp. 301-311.

However, it is still probable that in the human race a special differentiation has been established for the accomplishment of different and essential functions.

The organisation of human societies has certainly not followed the path by which social insects attained the formation of sexless individuals. It much more closely resembles what has taken place in some isolated animal types. A solitary bee, named *Halictus quadricinctus* (Fig. 27), is characterised by the fact that the female does not die when she has laid her last eggs, as generally happens amongst insects, but remains alive to cherish her offspring. This final portion of her life does not last long, and the bee cannot play the prominent part of governess in a society of insects organised by this specialisation of elderly females.

In the human race the individual life lasts longer and a division of labour takes place in the fashion suggested by *Halictus quadricinctus*.

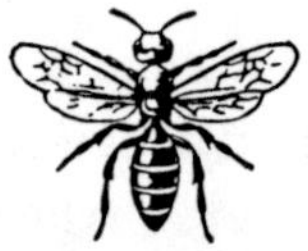

FIG. 27.—*Halictus quadricinctus.* (After Buffon.)

An ordinary woman ceases to be fertile at between forty and fifty years old, that is to say, at a time when, according to statistics, she has still on the average twenty years to live. During this long period, she can perform an extremely useful function in society, a function resembling that of the old mothers of *Halictus quadricinctus,* and consisting chiefly in the bringing up and education of the children. Who does not know the extraordinary devotion of grandmothers, and, as a general rule, of old women, who are extremely useful in bringing up children. And none the less, it must not be forgotten that, actually, old age begins too soon, that it is not what it ought to be under normal conditions, and that human life itself does not last nearly so long as it ought to do in ideal conditions. We may predict that when science occupies the preponderating place in human society that it ought to have, and when knowledge of hygiene is more advanced, human life will become much longer and the part of old people will become much more important than it is to-day.

The members of human society are not divided into sexual and neuter individuals as amongst insects, but the active life of every individual can be divided into two periods, the first one of productive activity, and the second of sterility but none the less devoted to work useful to the community. The essential difference between the two cases may be reduced to the contrast that whilst the individuals of which animal societies are composed are structurally incomplete, in human societies the individual preserves his integrity.

We come, then, to the result that the more highly organised a social being may be, so also the more highly developed is his individuality. It follows that amongst the theories which seek to control social life, those are the best which leave a field sufficiently wide and free for the development of individual initiative. The ideal which has been so often advocated and according to which the individual is to be sacrificed as completely as possible to society, cannot be regarded as in harmony with the general law of organic associations. Special conditions exist in social life in which great sacrifices are inevitable, but such an arrangement cannot be considered as general and permanent. We may predict that the more human beings succeed in advancing communal life, the fewer cases there will be in which the individual has to be sacrificed.

In the hope of subduing the egoism rooted in human nature, moralists have preached renunciation of individual happiness and the need of subordinating it to the good of the community. Very often such doctrine has borne little fruit, but there are cases where it has been embraced with such ardour that men and, still more, young women have been led to sacrifice their well-being for what they have taken to be the common good. However it may involve self-abnegation, there has been continued insistence on the duty of sacrificing the individual to the community.

The existing great inequalities in the distribution of wealth have revived doctrines the object of which is to redress such injustice. For more than a century, different forms of socialism have claimed to formulate rules for the amelioration of mankind. They agree in a verdict against existing conditions, but follow different paths in their proposals for the reformation of society. The varieties of socialism are so numerous that it is difficult even to define the word. Although collectivist theories have lost much of their early thoroughness, they are still far from admitting the just claims of the individuals constituting the society. At socialist assemblies and congresses the resolutions adopted frequently proclaim aggressively the sacrifice of the rights of the individual. The members of one socialist party have been seen refusing the collaboration of newspapers which are not the official organs of the party, or declining any co-operation with a government they have proscribed. In strikes organised by socialists, work is forbidden to men who ardently desire it. Recently printers have refused to set up newspapers the opinions of which they did not share, and even doctors have been known to decline to treat those belonging to another political party.

It is no new charge against collectivists that they would encroach too much on individual liberty. They reply that " in social-democratic society of the future, tyranny and oppression will be impossible. The secret of the bond will reside in a discipline totally different from the inanimate obedience of the soldier, a discipline depending on a willing submission of the individual to the group because of the common object."[1] But such discipline and submission may go so far that the conscience of the individual is seriously offended. And so amongst the socialists themselves there has arisen a small group which declines to accept this submergence of the individual in the whole. This group is composed of anarchists, who, in the name of liberty and the individual, attack the property and sometimes the lives of their opponents.

It appears that there has been a notable evolution of collectivist theories in the century or more in which the abolition of human misery has been an accepted problem. Whilst there was formerly advocated the total abolition of private property and the establishment of phalansteries for communal life, at the present time the demand is limited to the nationalisation of the means of production, leaving housing and food to be provided by individual property.

Through a publication, of M. Kautsky, one of their best known representatives, the social democrats have announced that "the nationalisation of the land does not necessarily bring with it the abolition of private dwellings. The customary attachment of the dwelling to agricultural employment will cease, but there is no reason why the peasants' houses should become collective property." "Modern socialism does not exclude individual property in food. One of the most important, perhaps the most important factor, in making human life happy and adding to its pleasures is the possible attainment of a private house. Collective owner-

[1] W. Herzberg, *Sozialdemokratie und Anarchismus*, 1906, p. 17.
[2] *Le problème agraire*, 1905, p. 147.

ship of the land does not exclude this." It is very difficult to separate house and garden, especially from the point of view of considering the pleasures of life. A garden furnishes the opportunity for endless improvements, many of which cannot be separated from the idea of individual property. The concessions which collectivists have been compelled to make show conclusively the importance of private property.

Notwithstanding such modifications, many voices have been raised against the prospect of the socialisation of the means of production and the concomitant limitations of individual enterprise. The great English philosopher, Herbert Spencer,[1] against whom narrowness of view or conservatism could be urged, energetically attacked collectivist doctrines as tending to reduce human individuality to a dead level. By a series of cogent instances, he showed the evil results of the best intentioned efforts to equalise opportunities and to abolish poverty. He foretold that slavery would be the real outcome if the State interfered too much in spheres that ought to be left to individual enterprise. He believed that the institution of a collectivist State would bring great dangers.

Nietzsche has attacked socialism with his customary exaggeration. "Socialism,"[2] he wrote, "is the fanatical younger brother of dying despotism, whose goods he wishes to inherit; his efforts are, in the deepest sense of the word, reactionary. He wishes a wealth of power in the State greater than despotism ever enjoyed, but he goes

[1] "The Coming Slavery" in *Man versus the State*, 1888, p. 18.
[2] *Human, too Human.* French translation, 1899, pp. 405-407. A German critic has reproached me for my ignorance of Nietzsche's works. I have read several of them, but the mixture of genius and madness in them makes them difficult to use. In this connection Moebius' volume, *Ueber das Pathologische bei Nietzsche* (Wiesbaden, 1902), is of interest.

beyond all the past inasmuch as he strives absolutely to stifle the individual; for him the individual is a useless efflorescence of nature to be tamed into a useful organ of the community." Further, "Socialism at least teaches brutally and convincingly the danger of concentrating power in the State, for it is a covert attack on the State itself. When its harsh voice raises the war-cry ' Let the State control as much as possible,' the cry will at first become louder; but soon another phrase will grow equally clamant, ' Let the State control as little as possible.' "

It is most probable that no shade of socialism will be able to solve the problem of social life with a sufficient respect for the maintenance of individual liberty. None the less the progress of human knowledge will inevitably bring about a great levelling of human fortunes. Intellectual culture will lead men to give up many things that are superfluous or even harmful, and that are still thought indispensable by most people. The conceptions that the greatest good fortune consists in the complete evolution of the normal cycle of human life and that this goal can be reached most easily by plain and sober habits will convince men of the folly of much of the luxury that now shortens human existence. Whilst the rich will choose a simpler mode of life and the poor will be able to live better, none the less, private property, acquired or inherited, may be maintained. Evolution must be gradual and much effort and new knowledge is required. Sociology, a new-born science, must learn of biology, her older sister. Biology teaches us that in proportion that the organisation becomes more complex, the consciousness of individuality develops, until a point is reached at which individuality cannot be sacrificed to the community. Amongst low creatures such as *Myxomycetes* and *Siphonophora*, the individuals disappear wholly or almost wholly in the community; but the sacrifice is small, as in these creatures the consciousness of individuality has not appeared. Social insects are in a stage intermediate between that of the lower animals and man. It is only in man that the individual has definitely acquired consciousness, and for that reason a satisfactory social organisation cannot sacrifice it on pretext of the common good. To this conclusion the study of the social evolution of living beings leads me.

It is plain that the study of human individuality is a necessary step in the organisation of the social life of human beings.

PART VII

PESSIMISM AND OPTIMISM

I

PREVALENCE OF PESSIMISM

Oriental origin of pessimism—Pessimistic poets—Byron—Leopardi—Poushkin—Lermontoff—Pessimism and suicide

In the attempt to formulate a pessimistic theory of human nature, we are naturally led to ask why it is that so many famous men have come to a purely pessimistic conception of human life.

Pessimism, although it has been most prominent in modern times, is extremely old. Everyone knows the pessimistic wail of Ecclesiastes, written nearly ten centuries before our era: "Vanity of Vanities, all is vanity." Solomon, the supposed author, states that he "hated life, because the work that is wrought under the sun is grievous unto me, for all is vanity and vexation of spirit" (Eccl. ii., 17).

Buddha raised pessimisim to the rank of a doctrine. All life seemed to him sorrow. "Birth is sorrow, old age is sorrow, disease is sorrow, union with one whom we do not love is sorrow, separation from one whom we love is sorrow, not to gratify desire is sorrow, in short, our five bonds with the things of the earth are sorrow."[1] This Buddhistic

[1] Quoted by Oldenberg, *Le Bouddha*, French translation, Paris, 1894, p. 214.

pessimism has been the source of most of the modern pessimistic theories.

Pessimism arose in the East and was much in vogue in India even apart from Buddhism. In the poems known under the name of Bhartrihari, and dating from the beginning of the Christian era, human life has been commiserated in the following fashion. "One hundred years are the limit of the life of man; night takes half of them, half of the other half is childhood and old age, the rest is filled with diseases, with separations and the misfortunes that come from them, with working for others and with wasting one's time. Where can happiness be found in an existence most like to the bubbles in broken water?" "Man's health is destroyed by every kind of care and disease. When fortune comes to him, evil follows as if by an open door. Death takes all human beings, one after the other, and they can offer no resistance to their fate. What is there assured amongst all that the mighty Brahma has created?"[1]

Pessimistic theories spread from the Asiatic East to Egypt and Europe. Three centuries before the Christian era, there arose the philosophy of Hegesias, which maintained that experience was generally deceptive and that enjoyment was quickly followed by satiety and disgust. According to him, the sum of pain surpassed the sum of pleasure in life, so that happiness was unattainable, and in reality never existed. It was vain to seek pleasure and happiness, as these could not be realised. It was better to try to be indifferent, dulling feeling and desire. In fact, life was no better than death, and it was often preferable to end it by suicide. Hegesias was called *Pisithanatos*, the adviser of death. "Listeners thronged around him, his doctrine spread rapidly, and his disciples, persuaded by his voice,

[1] P. Régnaud, "Le pessimisme brahmanique," in *Annales du Musée Guimet*, 1880, vol. i, pp. 110-111.

gave themselves to death. Ptolemy was perturbed by it, and fearing that the dislike of life would become contagious, closed the school of Hegesias and exiled its master."[1]

The pessimistic tendency sometimes appears in the writings of many Greek and Latin philosophers and poets. Seneca wrote: "The spectacle of human life is lamentable. New misfortunes overwhelm you before you have freed yourself from the old ones."[2]

It is in modern days, however, that there has been the greatest spread of pessimism.

Besides the philosophical theories of the last century, those of Schopenhauer, von Hartmann and Mailaender, which I discussed sufficiently in *The Nature of Man*, poets have formulated a pessimistic view of life. Even Voltaire was a pessimist in the following lines:

> Alas! what are the course and the goal of life?
> Only follies and then the darkness.
> Oh Jupiter! in creating us you made
> A heartless jest.

In *The Nature of Man* I described Byron's expression of his conception of the evils of human life. Soon after the death of the great English poet, a celebrated Italian poet, Giacomo Leopardi, sounded a note of abandoned pessimism.

Here are words which he addressed to his own heart[3]: "Be quiet for ever, you have beaten enough, nothing is worthy of your beating and the earth is not worthy of your sighs. Life is nothing but bitterness and weariness, there is nothing else in it. The world is nothing but mire. Repose from now onwards. Be in despair for ever. Destiny has given us nothing but death. Despise henceforth your-

---

[1] Guyau, *La Morale d'Epicure*, 4th edition, 1904, p. 116.
[2] *Ad Marciam*, chap. x.
[3] *Poésies et œuvres morales*, by Leopardi. Translated into French 1880, p. 49.

self and nature, and the shameful concealed power which decrees the ruin of all and the infinite variety of all."

Leopardi makes his readers witnesses of his distraction and his grief : " I shall study the blind truth "—he wrote in a poem dedicated to Charles Pépoli—" I shall study the blind fates of things mortal and immortal. Why humanity came into existence, and was burdened with pain and sorrow, to what final end destiny and nature are driving it, for whose pleasure or advantage is our great pain, what order, what laws rule this mysterious universe which wise men cover with praise, and I am content to wonder at " (*ibid.*, p. 15).

Quite a school of poets has been developed, singing the pain of the world, the " Weltschmerz " of German authors, amongst whom Heine and Nicolas Lenau are specially distinguished.

Russian poetry was born under the influence of Byronism, and its best exponents, Poushkin and Lermontoff, often laboured over the problem of the object of human existence, finding only sad answers. Poushkin, who is justly regarded as the father of lyric poetry in Russia, stated his pessimistic conception in the following lines :—

> Useless gift, gift of chance,
> Life, why wert thou given me?
> And why from the beginning art thou doomed
> Irrevocably to death?
>
> What unfriendly power
> Has drawn me from the darkness,
> Has filled my soul with passion,
> And breathed doubt into my soul?
>
> There is no goal for me,
> My heart and my soul are empty;
> And the dull emotion of life
> Has filled me with black care.

Recently, Mde. Ackermann, in a series of short poems, has given voice to the grief caused to her by the world and life as they are, although she does not state exactly the reason of her bitter complaints.

Whilst pessimistic philosophers and poets reflect the thoughts and feelings of their contemporaries, it is certain that they also seriously influence their readers. And so there has come into existence a deeply rooted conviction that the miseries of human life are far from being countervailed by its happiness. Probably such ideas have influenced the number of suicides. We do not know with any certainty the real motives of most cases of self-destruction, but it cannot be denied that the trend of modern thought has played an important part. According to statistics, the chief causes of suicide are "hypochondria, melancholia, weariness of life, and unbalancing of the mind." Thus from the Danish statistics it appears (and Denmark is the country in which suicide is most prevalent) that of 1,000 cases of suicides of males, between 1866 and 1895, 224, or one-quarter, were referred to the causes I have just mentioned. In the case of women, the corresponding figures are higher, amounting to nearly one-half (403 out of 1,000). The second most common cause of male suicides is alcoholism (164 in 1,000).[1] It is very probable that pessimism was the determining condition in most of the suicides referred to these two categories of causes. Leaving out of the question the true cases of mental alienation, amongst the victims of melancholia, hypochondria and weariness of life, in whom the mental condition was not pathological in the strict sense of the word, there must have been many who killed themselves because their view of life was pessimistic. And amongst the victims of drink, there are many who take to

[1] These facts are taken from Westergaard, 2nd edit., 1901, p. 649.

alcohol because they are convinced that life is not worth preserving.

The progressive increase in the numbers of suicides in modern times is an index of the great influence of pessimism. There have been even societies for the promotion of suicide. In such a society, founded in Paris in the beginning of last century, members placed their names in an urn, to be drawn by chance. He whose name was drawn had to kill himself in the presence of the other members. According to its rules, this society admitted only persons of honour who must have had experience of "the injustice of man, the ingratitude of a friend, the infidelity of a wife or mistress, and who, moreover, for many years had had a void in their souls and a distaste of what this world can offer."[1]

Although such societies no longer exist, individuals continue to put their lives to an end, in greater numbers every year.

[1] Dieudonné, *Archiv für Kulturgeschichte*, 1903, vol. i, p. 357.

II

ANALYSIS OF PESSIMISM

Attempts to assign reasons for the pessimistic conception of life—Views of E. von Hartmann—Analysis of Kowalevsky's work on the Psychology of Pessimism

In view of the facts I brought together in my last chapter, there is occasion to inquire if it be possible to discover the intimate mechanism by which men arrive at a conception of life as an evil to be got rid of as quickly as possible. Why do so many think that man is less happy than the beasts, and that cultured and intelligent men are more unhappy than those who are ignorant or feeble-minded?

I have related how in a society of friends of suicide, injustice and unfaithfulness were regarded as prime factors in arousing a distaste for life. Shakspeare made Hamlet exclaim that if it were possible to put an end to our days no one would continue to live:—

> For who would bear the whips and scorns of time,
> The oppressor's wrong, the proud man's contumely?

For Byron, besides diseases, death and slavery, the evils that we see, there are others:—

> And worse, the woes we see not—which throb through
> The immedicable soul, with heart-aches ever new.

In many of his works he insists on the feeling of satiety

which was almost continually upon him. Every sensation of pleasure that came to him was rapidly succeeded by a still stronger feeling of disgust.

Heine thought that existence was evil and saw

> . . . . across the hard surfaces of the rocks
> The homes of men and the hearts of men—
> In the one as in the others, lies, imposture and misery.

As I urged in *The Nature of Man*, consciousness of the shortness of human life has been an important factor in exciting pessimism, and we find this theme recurring in pessimistic writers. Leopardi returns to it again and again in his poems. " Falling in peril of death from some mysterious disease," he said in his *Souvenirs*, "I lamented over my sweet youth and the flower of my poor days which was to fall so soon, and often in the midnight hours wove from my sorrows, by the pale light of my lamp, a sad poem, and in the silence of the night wept over my fleeting life, and half fainting, sang to myself my funeral song " (*loc. cit.*, p. 28). The bas-relief on an ancient tomb, representing the departure of a young girl who took farewell of her friends, suggested to Leopardi the following thoughts : " Mother, who from their birth makes her family of living beings tremble and weep, Nature, monster unworthy of our praise, who brings into the world and nurtures only to kill, if the premature death of a mortal be evil, why do you bring it on so many innocent heads ? If it be a good, why do you make it sad for those who go and for those left behind ? Why is it the hardest grief to console ? The only relief from our woes is death, death, the inevitable end, the immutable law which you have established for human beings. Why, alas, after the sad voyage of life, do you not make the arrival joyful ? This certain end, this end which is in our souls all our lives, which alone can soothe our troubles,

ANALYSIS OF PESSIMISM

why do you drape it in black and surround it with mournful shades? Why do you make the harbour more terrible than the open seas?" (*loc. cit.*, p. 55).

The three chief grievances—injustice, disease, and death—often come together. From the anthropomorphic point of view fate is represented as a sort of wicked being who commits injustice by visiting all kinds of evils on mankind.

A pessimistic conception of life is arrived at by a complex psychological process in which both feelings and reflection are involved, and hence it is difficult to analyse it satisfactorily. Formerly, therefore, writers were content with general and very vague estimates of the process by which we may become pessimists. Ed. von Hartmann has tried to deal more exactly with this inner process of the human mind. In the first place, he lays stress on the fact that pleasures always bring less satisfaction than pains bring grief. False notes in music, for instance, are more painful than the best music is delightful. The pain of toothache is much more violent than the pleasure when relief comes. So also with all diseases. In love, according to Hartmann, the pleasure is always very greatly over-balanced by the pain. Muscular work brings pleasure only in a very small degree, and devotion to science and art and intellectual work in general brings more pain than pleasure to the votaries. As the result of an analysis, Hartmann is convinced that there is much more pain than pleasure in the world. Pessimism is founded upon the essential nature of human feelings.

M. Kowalevsky,[1] a German philosopher at Koenigsberg, adopting the modern habit of measuring mental processes as exactly as possible, has recently published an attempt

---

[1] Kowalevsky, *Studien zur Psychologie des Pessimismus*, Wiesbaden, 1904.

to analyse pessimism psychologically. Although this has not solved the problem, it is extremely interesting as an instance of the application of the methods now being adopted in modern psychology.

M. Kowalevsky took advantage of all the known methods of estimating the relative values of our emotions; he tried to make use of the notes of Munsterberg, another living psychologist who kept a journal in which he set down daily his psychical and psycho-physical impressions. The object of the work had no relation to the question of pessimism, and for that reason Kowalevsky thought that it was specially important in his investigations.

Munsterberg was not content with the existing classification of emotions as agreeable or painful. He subdivided them much further. He recognised, for instance, emotions of tranquillity and excitement, serious and pleasant impressions. Having completed the reckoning, Kowalevsky came to the conclusion that his colleague, who was by no means a pessimist, but a psychologist of well-balanced mind, experienced many more painful emotions (about 60 per cent. as compared with 40 per cent.) than agreeable emotions. "Such a result is in favour of pessimism," concluded Kowalevsky.

However, he went beyond the foregoing enquiry. By several other methods, he tried to gain an exact idea of the value of our emotions. He visited elementary schools in order to investigate the pleasures and pains of the scholars. In the case of 104 boys, of eleven to thirteen years of age, he found that pain was much more deeply felt than corresponding pleasure. Thus, while in 88 cases illness was set down as an evil, only in 21 was health reckoned as a good. One-third of the pupils noted down war amongst evils, whilst only one noted peace amongst the good things.

Poverty was written down thirteen times as an evil, against twice in which riches were put down as a good. In another series of investigations, Kowalevsky took notes on the pleasures and pains felt by pupils of the two sexes attending the same school. The result was that the greatest evil, according to them, was illness, noted 43 times, then death 42 times, after which came fire 37 times, hunger 23 times, floods 20 times. Amongst the good things, the first place was given, as might have been expected, to games (30) and the second to presents.

As Kowalevsky did not find that such investigations could solve the problem, he tried to discover a more exact method. With this object, he turned to different sensations, such as those of smell, hearing and taste, to which he applied methods of exact measurement. In the case of taste, for instance, he determined the minimum quantity of different substances which could excite definitely pleasant or unpleasant sensations. In his experiments, Kowalevsky found that doses which gave bad tastes were not balanced by those which gave good tastes. For instance, to neutralise the unpleasant taste of quinine, it was necessary to employ a much larger quantity of sugar. He was specially pleased with one experiment. Four persons were given definite mixtures of sugar and quinine in order to discover the proportion of the two substances necessary to obtain a neutral sensation. He found that to take away the bad taste of quinine, it was necessary to double the quantity of sugar given. Similarly with smells, he found that those which were unpleasant were appreciated much more strongly than those which were pleasant. Here, then, was a series of scientific results supporting the view of the pessimists. Must we really conclude from them that the world is very badly arranged? The analysis of good and bad temper made by Kowalevsky is in favour of such an interpretation. In order to estimate these conditions of mind, he measured the gait, that is to say, the number of steps taken in a minute. This method depended upon the following idea. It is an accepted view that the condition of mind is shown by the rapidity of the human walk; we have only to compare the slow pace of a man in deep grief with the rapid steps of a man in a state of joy. Pain, as a general rule, depresses, while joy stimulates voluntary movements. The result of the measurements taken according to this method give a new argument in favour of pessimism. However, it is useless to attempt to analyse these figures on which Kowalevsky had to employ the integral calculus, because the principle of his method cannot be supported. As a matter of fact, the rapidity of walking is an index of the degree of excitation, and not of the happy or unhappy condition of the mind. When a person suddenly undergoes a strong impression, either pleasant or unpleasant, he takes to walking actively about in his room, and may even want to go out of doors to walk more quickly. A letter which has been received and which gives some unexpected news, as for instance of the infidelity of a person one loves, or of an inheritance which one did not expect, produces a condition of excitement shown chiefly by rapid walking. Many orators and professors have to make gestures and to walk about in the course of their lectures. A man of science to whom some new idea comes and who wishes to think it out, rises from his chair and begins to walk. But not only on such pleasant occasions, but when one has to face an insult or an act of defiance which makes one very angry, the need to walk actively is felt. It is therefore impossible to utilise records of movements in the study of the pessimistic state of mind.

M. Kowalevsky employed still another mode of attacking the problem. He examined the recollection of painful or pleasant impressions. He asked the children of both sexes, whom he was investigating, questions which gave him indications as to whether pleasures or pains made the more lasting impression on the memory, and he registered the answers. The result, which agreed with what had already been obtained by Mr. Colegrove, an American psychologist, was unfavourable to the pessimistic view. He found, in fact, that in the majority of cases (70 per cent.) recollection of pleasant impressions predominated. However, in such investigations there is a facile source of error arising from the condition of mind of those who are being questioned. It is probable that Kowalevsky made his enquiry in school during recreation time, when most of the pupils were free from the boredom of the actual class. When we are happy the tendency exists in us to recall pleasant impressions of the past. If the enquiry had been made during a difficult or wearying lesson, or on children shut up in a hospital, or undergoing punishment, it is probable that the result would have been reversed.

It is evident that all such attempts to solve a problem so complex as that of pessimism, even by the so-called exact methods of physiological psychology, cannot lead to any convincing result. Thus Kowalevsky's different investigations led to contradictory conclusions. Whilst some of his series of facts supported the pessimistic conception, others were opposed to it, and he obtained no definite general conclusion. How can one expect to apply a method of measurement to sensations and emotions so different, not only from the qualitative point of view, but also in relation to their intensity? Take, for instance, the case of an individual who has experienced in one day nine sensations which were painful and one which was agreeable. According to the valuation of experimental psychologists, he ought to have reason to become a pessimist. However, this may be far from the case, if the nine painful impressions were much weaker than the single happy impression. The first were provoked by small wounds to his pride, fleeting pains of no importance, and small losses of money, whilst the happy emotion came from receiving a love letter. The sum of the ten impressions would be a happy one, and might well put him in an optimistic frame of mind. The learned attempts of experimental psychologists must be abandoned, as incapable of illuminating the problem. If, however, the human spirit still seeks some means of explaining the psychology of pessimism, there remains only the less subtle method given by the biographical study of human beings.

III

PESSIMISM IN ITS RELATION TO HEALTH AND AGE

>Relation between pessimism and the state of the health—History of a man of science who was pessimistic when young, and who became an optimist in old age—Optimism of Schopenhauer when old—Development of the sense of life—Development of the senses in blind people—The sense of obstacles

ANIMALS and children in good health are generally cheerful and of optimistic temperament. As soon as they fall ill they become sad and melancholy until their recovery. We may infer from this that an optimistic view is correlated with normal health, whilst pessimism arises from some physical or mental disease. And so in the case of the prophets of pessimism, we may seek for the origin of their views in some affliction. The pessimism of Byron has been attributed to his club-foot, and that of Leopardi to tuberculosis, these two nineteenth century exponents of pessimism having died whilst young. Buddha and Schopenhauer, on the other hand, reached old age, whilst Hartmann died when sixty-four years old. Their diseases at the time when they formed their theories could not have been very dangerous, and none the less they took a most gloomy view of human existence. The recent historical investigations of Dr. Iwan Bloch[1] make it very probable that Schopenhauer, in his youth, contracted syphilis. There

[1] *Medicinische Klinik*, 1906, n. 25 and 26.

has been found a note-book of the great philosopher in which he wrote down the details of the severe mercurial treatment which he had to undergo. The disease, however, was not contracted until several years after the appearance of his great pessimistic work.

Although we must attach due weight to the connection between disease and pessimism, we can assure ourselves that the problem is more complex than it appears at first sight. It is well known that blind people often enjoy a constant good humour, and, amongst the apostles of optimism, there has been the philosopher Duering,[1] who lost his sight during his youth.

Moreover, it has been noticed that persons affected with chronic diseases frequently have a very optimistic conception of life, whilst young people in full strength may become sad, melancholic, and abandoned to the most extreme pessimism. Such a contrast has been well described by Émile Zola in his novel *La Joie de Vivre*, where a rheumatic old man, tried by severe attacks of gout, maintained his good humour, whilst his young son, although vigorous and in good health, professed extreme pessimism.

I have a cousin who lost his sight in early youth. When he grew up he formed a most enviable judgment of life. He lived in his imagination and everything in life seemed to him good and beautiful; he married, and pictured his wife to himself as the most beautiful woman in the world, and thus he feared nothing more than the recovery of his sight. He had adapted himself to live without sight, and was convinced that the reality was much lower than his imagination. He feared that if he were able to see his wife she would appear to him less beautiful.

[1] *Der Werth des Lebens.*

I know a girl twenty-six years old, blind from her birth, the subject of infantile paralysis and liable to fits of epilepsy. She is nearly an idiot, lives in a carriage, and sees life from its best side. She is certainly the most happy member of all her family.

The good humour and megalomania of those affected with general paralysis of the insane also is well known. All such examples show that pessimism cannot be explained as depending on bad health.

Examination of the state of mind of a pessimist may throw some light on the subject. There has been within my own circle a typical case of a person who went through a phase of life in which everything seemed as gloomy as possible. My intimate knowledge of him makes it possible to apply my observations to the matter under discussion.

The subject was born of parents of good health and in comfortable circumstances, so that, from the beginning of his life, he was surrounded by a favourite environment. He lived in the country and escaped the diseases of childhood, so that he reached maturity in good health, and passed well through college and the university. Science attracted him, and he had the ambition to become a distinguished investigator. He threw himself into a scientific career with zeal and ability. His ardent disposition, although certainly favourable to work, was the cause of many troubles. He wished to succeed too quickly, and the obstacles he encountered embittered him. As he thought himself naturally talented, he conceived it to be the duty of his seniors to aid his development. And so, when he met with natural and very common indifference from those who had already become successful, the young man thought that there was a plot against him, to bring to nothing his scientific talents. From this view, many quarrels and difficulties arose, and as he could not overcome these sufficiently quickly, he fell into a mood of pessimism. In this life, he said to himself, the main thing is to adapt oneself to external conditions. According to Darwin's law of natural selection, the individuals who do not succeed in adapting themselves go to the wall. The survivors are not the best but only the most cunning. In the history of the earth it has been seen that many lower animals have long survived creatures much higher in organisation and general evolution. Whilst so many of the higher mammals, the nearest relatives of man, have been crushed out of existence, simpler animals, such as evil-smelling cockroaches, have survived from the remotest times, and multiply in the neighbourhood of man in despite of his efforts to exterminate them. The animal series and human evolution itself show that delicacy of the nervous system, with its concomitant extreme development of the sensibilities, hinders the power of adaptation and brings with it insuperable evils. The least blow to his pride, or a slighting word from a comrade, threw this pessimist into a most painful condition. No, he would cry, it would be better to be without friends, if one is to be wounded so deeply by them. It would be best to seclude oneself in some remote spot and be engrossed in one's work. He was very impressionable and a lover of music, and from his visits to the opera, he retained in his mind an air from the "Flûte enchantée." "Were I as small as a snail, I would hide myself in my shell." His moral hypersensibility was associated with physical hyperæsthesia. Noises of all kinds, such as the whistling of railway-trains, the cries of street-vendors, or the barking of dogs, excited extremely painful sensations. The least trace of light prevented him from sleeping at night. The unpleasant flavour of most drugs made it impossible for him to take medicine. He agreed thoroughly with the pessimistic philosophers who declare that the ills of life far surpass the good things. He required no experiments on the sense of taste to convince him. He believed that the organisation of his body prevented him from becoming adapted to external conditions and that he would have to disappear like the mammoth and the anthropoid apes.

The course of his life confirmed the convictions of our pessimist. He had no private fortune and married a woman who became affected with tuberculosis, and so was confronted with the greatest evils of existence. A young lady, hitherto in good health, contracted influenza in some northern town. It was a mere nothing, said the doctors; influenza is everywhere and no one escapes it; after a little patience and rest, she will be well again. However the "influenza" persisted and brought with it feebleness and wasting. The doctors then found that there was a little dullness in the apex of the left lung, but as there was no bad family history, there was nothing to fear. I need not describe the familiar course of events. The trifling influenza was replaced by degeneration of the left lung, and brought death after four years of great suffering. Towards the end, when there was no hope, the patient found her only solace in morphine. Under the influence of that drug, she passed hours free from pain and in relative calm, but her excited imagination passed almost into hallucination.

It is not surprising that the death of his wife was a severe shock to the husband. His pessimism became complete. He was a widower at the age of twenty-eight years, and, in his condition of mental and physical exhaustion, took to morphine like his wife. He knew that it was a poison which would complete the ruin of his constitution and make his work impossible. But what was the value of his life? As his organisation was too nervous for him to adapt himself to external conditions, was it not as well to come to the aid of natural selection and so make room for others? As it happened, a large dose of morphia did not solve the problem. It produced in him a condition of extraordinary happiness combined with extreme physical weakness. Little by little the instinct of life awoke in him, and he resumed his work. Pessimism, however, remained the fundamental quality in his character. Life was not worth the pains necessary to protect it. It would be a true crime to bring into the world other living beings doomed to elimination by natural selection. Moral and physical sensibility, as they continued to develop, brought with them so much evil that there could be no good end. The "injustice" of those who were unwilling to "understand" him made life painful to the man himself and to those about him. The closest absorption and hard work made his existence more tolerable, but his pessimistic conception was not in the least altered. Thus, he was easily driven to morphia for consolation, when he suffered from some act of "injustice" or vexation. A severe fit of poisoning, however, stopped this excess.

Years passed. When he discussed with his friends the problem of the goal of human life and similar topics, he was always ardent in supporting the point of view of pessimism. However, he occasionally wondered if his pleading for this were really sincere. As his nature was honest and frank, this question which he put to his conscience appeared most curious to him. Analysis of what passed in his mind revealed to him a change. It was not that his conceptions had changed in the course of years, but rather his feelings and sensations. As he was now in full maturity, between forty-five and fifty years old, he found that there was a great change in the intensity of these last. Disagreeable sounds did not trouble him to the same extent as formerly, and he was undisturbed by the caterwauling of cats or by harsh street cries. As his hypersensibility diminished his character became more tolerant. Even the injustices or wounds to his pride which formerly drove him to morphia, no longer provoked in him any painful reaction. He could easily conceal the bad effect of these upon him, and no longer felt them with the same intensity. Thus his character had become much more supportable to those with him, and much better balanced.

"It is old age which is come upon me," he cried; "I feel painful impressions much less acutely and pleasant impressions have less effect on me. The relative proportions of the two remain as before, that is to say, unpleasant things still impress me much more strongly than pleasant things." By analysing and comparing his emotions, he discovered something new, in fact that some impressions were, so to speak, neutral. As he was less sensitive to unharmonious sounds, and at the same time less affected by music itself, he found himself in a more tranquil condition. Awakening in the middle of the night, he experienced a kind of happiness which reminded him of that formerly produced by morphine, and which was characterised by his hearing no sound, either pleasant or unpleasant. He became less disgusted by drugs, but at the same time indifferent to the pleasures of the table which he had appreciated in his youth. He also delighted in consuming more and more simple food. A piece of black bread and a glass of water became real treats to him. Insipid dishes, which he formerly despised, were now specially agreeable to him.

Just as in the evolution of art, violent coloration has yielded to the low tones of Puvis de Chavannes, as views of fields and meadows are preferred to those of mountains and lakes; just as in literature, tragic and romantic studies have been successfully replaced by scenes of daily life, so the psychical development of my friend displayed a similar change. Instead of taking his pleasure in mountains or in places famed for their picturesqueness, he was content to watch the budding of the leaves of the trees of his garden, or a snail overcoming its fears and putting out its horns. The simplest occurrences, such as the lisping or the smile of a baby or the first words of a child, became sources of real delight to this elderly man of science. What was the meaning of these changes which took so many years to be accomplished? It was the growth of his sense of life. The instinct of life is little developed in youth. Just as a young woman gets more pain than pleasure from the earlier part of her married life, just as a new-born baby cries, so the impressions from life, especially when they are very keenly felt, bring more pain than pleasure during a long period of human life. The sensations and feelings are not stable; they undergo evolution, and when that takes place more or less normally, it brings about a state of psychical equilibrium.

And thus my friend, formerly so entrenched in pessimism, came to share my optimistic view of life. The discussions that we had had for so many years ended in complete agreement. "However," said he, "to understand the value of life, one must have lived long; otherwise one is in the position of a man blind from his birth to whom are recounted the beauties of colours." In a word, my friend towards the end of his life changed from abject pessimism to complete optimism.

Such a transformation or evolution cannot be regarded as unusual. In *The Nature of Man*, I showed that most of the great pessimistic writers had been young men.

Such were Buddha, Byron, Leopardi, Schopenhauer, Hartmann, and Mailaender, and there might be added many other names of less well known men.

The question has often been asked why Schopenhauer, who was certainly sincere in his philosophy and who extolled Nirvana as the perfect state, came to have a strong attachment to life, instead of putting it to a premature end as was done later on by Mailaender. The reason was that the philosopher of Frankfort lived long enough to acquire a strong instinct of life. M. Moebius,[1] a well-known authority on madness, has made a close investigation of Schopenhauer's biography, and has established the fact that towards the end of his life his views were tinged with optimistic colours. On his seventieth anniversary, he took pleasure in the consoling idea of the Hindoo Oupanischad and of Flourens that the span of man's life might reach a century. As Moebius put it, " Schopenhauer as an old man enjoyed life and was no longer a pessimist" (p. 94). Not long before his death he still hoped to survive yet another twenty years. It is true that Schopenhauer never recanted his early pessimistic writings, but that was probably because he did not fully realise his own mental evolution.

In looking through the work of modern psychologists, I cannot find recognition of the cycle of evolution of the human mind. In Kowalevsky's able and conscientious study of pessimism, I was specially struck by one phrase. " Evils such as hunger, disease, and death are equally terrible at all stages of life and in every rank of society" (p. 95) said that author. I notice here a failure to recognise the modification of the emotions in the course of life which, none the less, is one of the great facts of human

[1] *Ueber Schopenhauer*, Leipzig, 1899.

nature. Fear of death is by no means equally great at all stages of life. A child is ignorant of death and has no conscious aversion from it. The youth and the young man know that death is a terrible thing, but they have not the horror of it that comes to a mature man in whom the instinct of life has become fully developed. And we see that young men are careless of the laws of hygiene, whilst old men devote to them sedulous attention. This difference is probably a notable cause of pessimism in young men. In his studies of the mind, Moebius[1] has stated his view that pessimism is a phase of youth which is succeeded by a serener spirit. "One may remain a pessimist in theory," he says, "but actually to be one, it is necessary to be young. As years increase, a man clings more firmly to life." "When an old man is free from melancholia, he is not a pessimist at heart." "We cannot yet explain clearly the psychology of the pessimism of the young, but at least we can lay down the proposition that it is a disease of youth" (p. 182).

The cases of Schopenhauer and of the man of science whose psychical history I have sketched fully confirm the view of the alienist of Leipzig.

The conception that there is an evolution of the instinct of life in the course of the development of a human being is the true foundation of optimistic philosophy. It is so important that it should be examined with the minutest care. Our senses are capable of great cultivation. Artists develop the sense of colour far beyond the point attained by ordinary men, and distinguish shades that others do not notice. Hearing, taste, and smell also can be educated. Wine tasters have an appreciation of wine much more acute than that of other men. A friend of mine, who does not

[1] Moebius, *Goethe*, vol. i, Leipzig, 1903.

PESSIMISM AND HEALTH AND AGE

drink wine, can distinguish burgundy from claret only by the shapes of the bottles, but is devoted to tea and has a very fine palate for different blends. I do not know if a good palate is a natural gift, but however this may be, it is certain that the palate can be brought to a high condition of perfection.

The development of the senses is specially notable in the case of the blind in whom other powers become extremely acute. As I thought that investigation of the educability of other senses in blind persons very important from the point of view of the development of the sense of life, I have tried to obtain the best available information on the question. The perfection of touch in the blind is accepted so generally as a truth that one would have expected to find convincing facts in its favour. However, it is not true. Griesbach,[1] using a well-known method for estimating tactile discrimination, found that the sense of touch is not more acute in the blind than in normal persons. Blind persons distinguished the points of a pair of compasses as separate, only when they were at least as far apart as in case of normal persons. Dr. Javal,[2] a well-known oculist who himself became blind, stated his surprise at finding that "tactile discrimination is quite notably less acute in the case of the blind than in the case of those with unimpaired vision. For instance, the index finger of a blind man who was a great reader got separate sensations from the points of a pair of compasses only when these were three millimetres apart, whilst a man with normal sight had the double sensation at a distance of two millimetres" (p. 123). Griesbach goes still farther, stating that neither hearing

[1] V. Kunz, "Zur Blindenphysiologie," *Wiener medicin. Wochenschrift*, 1902, No. 21.
[2] *Physiologie de la Lecture et de l'Écriture*, Paris, 1905.

nor smell is better developed in the blind than amongst normal people. Although these senses may come to replace to a certain extent the sense of sight, this occurs merely because the blind person uses impressions which the clear-sighted person hardly notices. As we see what is going on around us, we do not concentrate our attention on the different sounds and smells or other such phenomena. The blind person, on the other hand, not being absorbed by impressions of sight, gives attention to the others. Such and such a sound tells him that the garden gate of his neighbour has been opened to let out a carriage which he must avoid. A particular smell lets him recognise the place where he is, as stable or kitchen.

From the present point of view, it is not exactly the acuteness of the senses which is most important. The acuteness might be equal in a blind person and in a normal person. It might even be greater in the latter, and yet it is only the blind person who can decipher without difficulty raised points so as to understand their meaning as well as when a normal person reads a printed book. This power of the blind person is developed only after a long period of learning, and depends on the appreciation of very delicate tactile impressions. I must point out, moreover, that the method of deciding by means of a pair of compasses gives information only with regard to one side of the tactile sense.

However, although we admit that blind people do not really gain anything in the four remaining senses, there is developed in them a special kind of sensibility, which is spoken of in their case as a sixth sense, the "sense of obstacles." Blind people, especially those who have lost their sight in youth, acquire a surprising habit of avoiding obstacles and of recognising at a distance objects round about them. Blind children, for instance, can play in a garden, without knocking themselves against the trees.

Dr. Javal[1] states that some blind people, when passing in front of a house, can count the ground floor windows. A professor, who had been blind from the age of four years, could walk in the garden without striking against a tree or post. He appreciated a wall at a distance of two metres from it. One day, going for the first time into a large apartment, he recognised the presence of a big piece of furniture in the middle, which he took to be a billiard table.

Another blind man, walking in the street, could distinguish houses from shops and could count the number of doors and windows. The existence of this sense of obstacles rests upon so many exact facts that it is indubitable. The opinions as to the mechanism by which it operates, however, are very varied. Dr. Zell[2] thinks that it is not a sense peculiar to blind people and "that those of normal sight could equally well acquire it by practice, because it exists in nearly everyone without being noticed." None the less, there are some blind people who, even in the course of years, do not acquire it. M. Javal, for instance, learnt to read with his fingers extremely well, but was never able to distinguish obstacles at a distance.

The most probable hypothesis refers this sixth sense to the action of the tympanic membrane and the auditory apparatus. It is known that loud noise makes it more difficult to perceive obstacles, and snow, by dulling the sound of steps, has a precisely similar effect. Blind tuners, in whom the sense of hearing is well developed, have the sixth sense very marked.

The examples I have given show that the human body possesses senses which come into operation only in special

[1] *Entre aveugles*, Paris, 1903.   [2] *Der Blindenfreund*, Feb. 15th, 1906.

conditions, and which require a special education. The "sense of life" to a certain extent comes within this category. In some persons it develops very imperfectly, generally revealing itself only late in life, but sometimes a disease or the danger of losing life stimulates its earlier development. Occasionally in persons who have tried to commit suicide, a strong instinct of life wakens suddenly, and impels them to make frantic efforts to escape.

It happens, therefore, that the sense of life develops sometimes in healthy people, sometimes in those who suffer from acute or chronic disease. These variations are parallel with the development of the sexual instinct, which in some women is completely absent and in others develops only very late. In certain cases, it is awakened only by special conditions, such as child-birth, or even some defect of health.

As the sense of life can be developed, special pains ought to be taken with it, just as with the making perfect of the other senses in the blind. Young people who are inclined to pessimism ought to be informed that their condition of mind is only temporary, and that according to the laws of human nature it will later on be replaced by optimism.

PART VIII

GOETHE AND FAUST

I

GOETHE'S YOUTH

Goethe's youth—Pessimism of youth—Werther—Tendency to suicide—Work and love—Goethe's conception of life in his maturity

THERE can be drawn from analysis of the lives of great men information that is very important in the study of the constitution of man. I have chosen Goethe for several reasons. He was a man of genius distinguished by the comprehensive character of his ability. He was a poet and dramatist of the highest rank, his mind was stored with the most varied knowledge, and he contributed to the advancement of natural science. As minister of state and as the director of a theatre, he was occupied with practical affairs. He reached the age of eighty-three years, and he passed through the phases of life in relatively normal circumstances; in his many writings there are most valuable facts which throw a keen light on his life and nature. The Goethe cult in Germany has brought about the existence of fuller biographical details than exist regarding any other great man. He aspired to lead "the higher life," and, throughout his existence, he occupied himself with the most serious problems of humanity.

It is not surprising that Goethe became a subject of

investigation for me, but as the main facts as to his history are widely known I need not elaborate them here.

Goethe was reared in circumstances that were favourable in every respect, and from his earliest years showed remarkable traits. As his memory was good and his imagination vast, the study of ancient and modern languages and the routine curriculum of a classical education were little more than an amusement to him. The rich library of his father placed all sorts of books at his disposal, and whilst he was still young he devoted himself to reading with the enthusiasm and passion that were the chief qualities of his character. When he was fifteen years old he began to write verses, although he was still unconscious of his destiny as a poet. He intended to be a learned man, and looked forward to the career of a professor.

At the age of sixteen, he entered the University of Leipzig with the intention of studying natural science seriously. Law and philosophy interested him but little; he turned to natural science and medicine, although his actual study was rather superficial. His disposition was lively and restless; he made many friends, frequented the theatre and plunged into all kinds of gaiety. Extracts from letters he wrote during this period show the kind of life he led. When he was a student, eighteen years old, he wrote to a friend, " And so good-night; I am drunk as a hog." A month later, to the same friend, he summed up his life as a "delirium in the arms of Jetty."

He graduated in law at Strassburg, and became a barrister, but realising that such a career was unsuitable, he became a man of letters, encouraged by the success of his first literary efforts.

From the point of view of a writer, he sought all kinds of experiences. He devoted himself to literature and science, including even the occult sciences, and frequented the theatre and society. He was specially attracted by the imaginative side and gave little thought to the problems of science. "I must have movement," he wrote in one of his note-books.

When he was young, his temper was violent and he fell into fits of passionate rage. His contemporaries have related that when he was in such a condition he would destroy the illustrations and tear up the books on his work-table. These experiences have been vividly described in his famous romance, *The Sorrows of Werther*. I shall give a few extracts to show the exact state of mind of the young pessimist. "It is the fate of some men not to be understood." "Human life is a dream; I am not the first to say that, but the idea haunts me. When I reflect on the narrow limits which circumscribe the powers of man, his activities and intelligence; when I see how we exhaust our forces in satisfying our wants and that these wants are for no more than the prolongation of a miserable existence; that our acquiescence in so much is merely resignation engendered by dreams, like that of a prisoner who has covered the walls of his cell with pictures and new landscapes; such things, my friend, plunge me into silence." "Our learned teachers all agree that children do not know why they have desires; but that grown men should move on the earth like children, and, like these, be ignorant whence they have come and whither they go, like these strive little for real things, but be ruled by cakes and sweets and rods; no one will believe such things, though their truth is patent. I admit readily (for I know what you will say) that they are the happiest men who live from day to day like children, who play with their dolls, dress them and undress them, who reverence the cupboard where mamma keeps the gingerbread, and who, when they have got what they wish, cry, with their mouths full, 'How happy we are!'"

Werther proclaimed his pessimism before his romance with Charlotte, and it was his view of life that made his love-affair turn out unhappily. But the fame of Goethe's *Werther* was due, not to the tragic fate of the young lover, but to the general views which were in harmony with the conception of the world held by the best minds of the time. Byronism was born before Byron.

Werther affords a good illustration of the disharmonies in the development of man's psychical nature. Inclination and desires develop extremely strongly and before will. Just as in the development of the reproductive functions, as I showed in *The Nature of Man*, the different factors develop unequally and unharmoniously, so there is inequality and disharmony in the order of the appearance of the higher psychical faculties. Sexual appreciation and a vague attraction to the other sex appear at a time when there can be no possibility of the normal physical side of sex, with the result that many evils come about in the long period of youth. The precocious development of sensibility brings about a kind of diffused hyperæsthesia which may lead to trouble. The infant wishes to lay hold of everything he sees before him; he stretches out his arms to grasp the moon and suffers from his inability to gratify his desires. In youth there is still well-marked disharmony. Young people cannot realise the true relations of things, and formulate their desires before they understand that their will-power is not strong enough to gratify them, as will is the latest of the human powers to develop.

Werther fell in love with a kindred spirit and gave way to his passion without consideration of the difficulties, Charlotte being already betrothed to another. This is the plot of the tragedy of the young man, who committed suicide, having given way to pessimism. He had not the will-power to conquer his sentiments and so fell into a state of lassitude, until, weary of life, he could see no other end than to blow out his brains.

I need not linger over the last phase of the story of Werther, for it is the character of Goethe himself that is of interest. Goethe was able to subdue his passion for Lotte, and, after many amorous woes, consoled himself with another woman. Notwithstanding this difference, it is certain that in *Werther*, Goethe was telling part of the story of his own youth. Goethe himself is a witness to this, for in a letter to Kestner he wrote that " he was at work on the artistic reproduction of his own case." The letter was written in July, 1773, whilst Goethe, then a writer twenty-four years old, was relating the sorrows of young Werther.

The general tendency of *Werther* has been described excellently by Carlyle.[1] " *Werther*," he wrote, " is but the cry of that dim, rooted pain, under which all thoughtful men of a certain age were languishing; it paints the misery, it passionately utters the complaint; and heart and voice, all over Europe, loudly and at once responded to it." *Werther* was " the first thrilling peal of that impassioned dirge which, in country after country, men's ears have listened to, till they were deaf to all else."

In the pessimistic period of his life, Goethe often cherished the idea of suicide. In his biography he relates that at this time he used to have, by his bedside, a poisoned dagger, and that he had repeatedly tried to plunge it in his bosom. Of these times he wrote to his friend Zelter[2]—" I know

---

[1] *Critical and Miscellaneous Essays*, vol. i, pp. 164-5, in the Essay on Goethe.
[2] *Briefwechsel zwischen Goethe und Zelter.* Letter of Dec. 3, 1812.

what it has cost me in effort to resist the waves of death." The suicide which was the subject of the end of his romance made a deep impression upon him. Although he overcame his passion for Charlotte, his view of life remained tinged with pessimism for many years; in a note-book of 1773, for instance, he wrote " I am not made for this world."[1] These words are the more striking as they date from a period when exact ideas regarding the adaptation of the organism and the character to the environment did not exist. Goethe, with his too delicate sensibility, felt himself out of harmony with his environment.

It is very interesting to trace Goethe's subsequent development and the transformation of a youthful pessimist into a convinced optimist. Goethe found a remedy for his crises of grief in work, poetical creation and love. He declared that the mere describing his woes on paper brought assuagement. The tears that they shed console women and children; and the poetry in which he expresses his suffering consoles the poet. Goethe's romance with Charlotte was not quite at an end when he found himself ready to love her sister Helen. He wrote to Kestner in December, 1772:—" I was about to ask you if Helen had arrived, when I got the letter telling me of her return." " To judge from her portrait she must be charming, even more charming than Charlotte. Well, I am free and I am thirsting for love." " I am here at Frankfort again with new plans and new dreams, and all will be well if I find someone to love." Soon afterwards, in another letter to Kestner, he wrote:—" Tell Charlotte that I have found here a girl whom I love with all my heart; if I wanted to marry, I should choose her before anyone else."

As he had not yet realised his true vocation, Goethe became a court minister at Weimar. He devoted himself

[1] Quoted in Moebius' *Goethe*, vol. ii, p. 80.

to his duties with an enthusiasm that carried him far beyond the usual affairs of state. He wished to deepen his knowledge of such administrative problems as the construction of roads and the management of mines, and he studied geology and mineralogy with a real zest. Forest adminis tration and agriculture led him seriously into botany, and as he had the direction of a school of design, he thought it necessary to learn anatomy. Such varied work gave him a real taste for science. It was no longer the superficial interest that characterised his work at Leipzig and Strassburg but a true devotion which led him to important discoveries, some of which have become classic.

Even such varied occupations did not absorb his prodigious genius. In his leisure he wrote poetry and prose. Engrossed in so much work, he was happy. His discovery of the human intermaxillary bone suffused him with joy. His intense activity was strengthened by his love for Madame von Stein, a love that he declared was " a life-belt supporting him in the sea." A few hours with her in the evenings set free his soul.

The powerful influence of love on the life of Goethe was specially prominent in this period when he was passing from pessimistic youth to optimistic maturity. Being forced to separate from Madame von Stein, he gave way to grief that plunged him again in the worst hours of his life. At the age of thirty-seven he fell back into a crisis like that of the days of *Werther*. " I have discovered," he said in 1786, " that the author of *Werther* would have done well to blow out his brains when he had finished his work." Soon afterwards he wrote that " death would have been better than the last years of his life."

This relapse into pessimism was shorter and less acute than his first experience. He began to find that frequently his delight in existence and sense of life were proved by his fear of death. When he was little more than thirty years old, he began to take precautions against the chance of his death. He wrote to Lavater:—" I have no time to lose; I am already getting on in years, and it may be that fate will destroy me in the midst of my life." On all sides his wish to live and his shrinking from death reveal themselves. It was at this time, a few days after his thirty-first birthday, that he wrote those famous lines, counted amongst the finest of his poetry, on the summit of the Gickelhahn, on the wall of a small room, and which end with the presentiment of his own death, " Before long, you also will be at rest."

The crisis through which he passed at the age of thirty-seven, as the immediate result of his separation from Madame von Stein, but perhaps also partly due to brain fatigue, brought about his sudden departure from Weimar and his long sojourn in Italy. There he came to life again, and everything interested him, archæology, art and nature. The joy of life came back to him, and he soon consoled himself for the lost love of the blue-stocking Baroness in the arms of a pretty, blue-eyed girl of Milan. This girl, whose name was Maddalena Riggi, like Charlotte, was already betrothed, a circumstance, however, that had a different result. Even after she had given up the man to whom she had been engaged, Goethe avoided any permanent bond and soon abandoned her definitely. He chose to associate with Faustine, another Italian girl, with whom he lived during the last period of his stay at Rome. This affair, which was less ideal and much simpler than his love for Madame von Stein, he has described in his *Roman Elegies*, which throw a vivid light on his temperament. I shall give some characteristic extracts.

" A sacred enthusiasm inspires me on this classic soil; the old world and the world around me raise their voices and draw me to them. Here I follow the ideas and turn over the pages of the ancient writers, giving myself no rest whilst day lasts and ever reaching new delights. By night love calls me to other cares; and if I am only half a philosopher, I am twice happy. But may I not say that I am also learning when my eye follows the contours of a loving breast, when with my hand I trace the lines of her form? It is then that I understand marble, I think and compare, I see with an eye that touches and touch with a hand that sees." "Often I have made verses in her arms; often my playful finger has softly beaten out my hexameters on her back. As she breathes in her sweet sleep, her breath burns me to my innermost soul." [1]

His stay in Italy brought Goethe definitely to maturity. On this important stage in his life let us hear his biographer, Bielschowsky. "The voyage to Italy made a new man of him. His sickliness and nervousness disappeared. The melancholy which led him to think of early death and made him regard death as better than the former conditions of his life was replaced by a sublime serenity and joy in living. The taciturn and preoccupied man who in no society abandoned his grave thoughts had become happy as a child" (vol. i, p. 412). "From this time on, in calm and enviable security, he passed through the cycle of life which seemed so mysterious to others. Goethe became the serene Olympian, the wonder of posterity, whilst many of his contemporaries no longer saw in him the passionate pilgrim" (*ibid.*, p. 417).

It was after reaching the age of forty years that Goethe entered on the optimistic phase of his life.

---

[1] *The Fifth Roman Elegy*, Blaze's French translation, 1873 p. 186. Some of Goethe's biographers, and amongst them G. H. Lewes, maintain that these lines relate to Christine, Goethe's wife. This is erroneous; they refer to Faustine (see Bielschowsky, i, p. 517).

II

GOETHE AND OPTIMISM

Goethe's optimistic period—His mode of life in that period—Influence of love in artistic production—Inclinations towards the arts must be regarded as secondary sexual characters—Senile love of Goethe—Relation between genius and the sexual activities

THE moral equilibrium of the great writer was not established once for all. In the course of his life, Goethe had several relapses into pessimism which, however, were ephemeral, and after which he became a man as complete and harmonious as was possible in the circumstances of his life. He reached a serene old age, and his activity did not relax until after his eightieth year, when he died.

As I have already said, Goethe realised the value of life in good time. Having become an optimist, he experienced the joy of existence and coveted as much of it as possible. When he was an old man, he declared that life, like the Sibylline books, became more valuable the fewer of them were left. There appeared in him a normal phase of human nature. The conditions under which he lived, however, were far from ideal. His health was indifferent. In his youth he suffered from severe hæmorrhage, probably tuberculous, and throughout his life he was subject to various more or less serious maladies, such as gout, colic, nephritis, and intestinal troubles. His habits were unwholesome. He was brought up in a region of vineyards, and in his youth he acquired the habit of drinking wine in quantities certainly harmful. This he himself realised, and when he was thirty-one years old, after he had acquired the instinct of life, he gave it serious attention. "I wish I could abstain from wine," he wrote in his note-book. Some weeks later he wrote, "I now drink almost no wine."[1]

But he had not the strength of character to remain temperate, and soon after his decision, he had fits of bleeding at the nose, which he attributed to "having taken some glasses of wine."[2] To his last day, he took wine regularly, and sometimes to excess. J. H. Wolff, who dined with him at Weimar, when he was in his eightieth year, was surprised by his appetite and by the quantity of wine he drank. "In addition to other food, he ate an enormous portion of roast goose, and drank a bottle of red wine."[3] In Eckermann's interesting narrative of the last ten years of Goethe's life (1822—1832) there is repeated mention of wine. Goethe seized every occasion to drink it. Sometimes it was the visit of a stranger, sometimes a present of some famous vintage. It was said that he drank from one to two bottles of wine daily (Moebius). None the less, he was convinced that wine was not good for intellectual work. He had remarked that when his friend Schiller had drunk more than usual, to increase his strength and stimulate his literary activity, the result was deplorable. He said to Eckermann (March 11, 1828), "He will ruin his health and will spoil his work. That is why he has made the faults the critics have pointed out." In another conversation (March 11, 1828) he stated that what was written

---

[1] Moebius' *Goethe*, vol. ii, pp. 84-87.
[2] Moebius' *Goethe*, vol. ii, pp. 84-87.
[3] Quoted by Bode in *Goethe's Lebenskunst*, Berlin, 1905, p. 59.

under the influence of wine was abnormal and forced, and ought to be deleted.

Love was the great stimulus of Goethe's genius. The love affairs, the histories of which fill his biography, are well known. Many have been shocked by them; others have tried to justify them. It has been suggested that his disposition made it necessary for him to impart his ideas and obtain sympathy for them, and that his love for women was the expression of a purely artistic feeling and had nothing in common with the ordinary passion.

The truth is that artistic genius and perhaps all kinds of genius are closely associated with sexual activity. I agree with the proposition formulated by Dr. Moebius[1] that "artistic proclivities are probably to be regarded as secondary sexual characters." Just as the beard and some other male characters are developed as means of attracting the female sex, so also bodily strength, strong voice and many of the talents must be regarded as due to the need to fulfil the sexual relations. In primitive conditions woman worked more than man; man's superior force served him principally in fighting with other males, the object of the combats usually being possession of a woman. Just as a victorious combatant covets the presence of a woman as witness of his prowess, so an orator speaks better in the presence of a woman to whom he is devoted. Singers and poets are stimulated in their arts by the love they awaken. Poetic genius is intimately associated with sexual power and castration inhibits it. Just as castrated animals retain their physical strength, but become changed in character, losing in particular their combative nature, so a man of genius loses much of his quality with the sexual function. Amongst the eunuchs on record, Abelard is the only poet,

[1] *Ueber die Wirkungen d. Castration*, Halle, 1903, p. 82.

but Abelard was forty years old when he ceased to be a man, and at the same time he ceased to be a poet. Many singers have been eunuchs, but they have been merely executants, and have taken no part in musical creation. Some musical composers have been eunuchs, but these were of mediocre ability and their names have been forgotten. When castration has taken place at an early age, it has a much more powerful influence in modifying the secondary sexual characters.

From the point of view of a naturalist, I cannot agree with the moralists who have blamed Goethe for his sexuality, nor do I share the views of those defenders of him who have wished to deny the facts or to explain them away by the suggestion that they did not relate to sexual love.

Extracts from the *Roman Elegies* show quite clearly what was the nature of Goethe's love affairs. His feelings towards the Baroness von Stein have been taken as revealing merely idealistic love. But some of his letters to her are clear evidence that their relations were erotic (Moebius, *Goethe,* vol. ii, p. 89). The love which he bore for Minna Herzlieb, the girl who inspired him to write *Elective Affinities* (*Wahlverwandschaften*), has been described by Goethe himself in a poem so crudely erotic that it has been impossible to publish it (Lewes, vol. ii, p. 314).

A fact to which I specially desire to call attention is that Goethe's amorous temperament survived until the end of his life, and all the world has been astonished by the vigour of his poetic genius in extreme old age.

Goethe has been the subject of derision because at the age of seventy-four years he fell deeply in love with Ulrique de Lewetzow, who was quite a young girl. This incident, however, merits close attention as it is a typical case of senile love in a man of genius.

Whilst he was at Carlsbad, Goethe became acquainted with a pretty girl seventeen years old, with beautiful blue eyes, brown hair, and of an ardent, good-humoured and happy disposition. In the first two seasons nothing in particular happened. But in the third summer, at Marienbad, Goethe became passionately enamoured of Ulrique, who was then nineteen years old and in the full bloom of her young womanhood. His love made him young again; he passed long hours with her and took to dancing with her. "I am quite certain," he wrote to his son, "that it is many years since I have enjoyed such health of body and mind" (Aug. 30, 1823). His passion became so serious that the Grand Duke of Saxe-Weimar, on behalf of his friend, made a formal proposal of marriage for Mademoiselle de Lewetzow. The mother gave an evasive answer, and the matter rested in suspense for long, and ended in a refusal. Goethe withdrew to his family, but encountered there strong opposition to his project of marriage.

This misadventure troubled the old poet so seriously that he fell ill. He suffered from pain in the region of the heart and from profound mental disturbance. He complained to Eckermann "that he could do nothing, that he could get to work on nothing, and that his mind had lost its power." "I can no longer work," he said. "I cannot even read, and it is only in rare and fortunate moments that I can think, feeling myself partially soothed" (Eckermann, Nov. 16, 1823). Eckermann makes the following reflection on the state of mind of the great old man. "His trouble seems to be not merely physical. The passionate desire which he acquired for a young lady at Marienbad this summer, and against which he is still struggling, must be regarded as the chief cause of his illness" (Nov. 17, 1823).

As in all earlier crises, Goethe sought consolation in poetry and love. He left Marienbad in a carriage and began to set down verses astonishingly vigorous for so old a man. His Marienbad elegy is held to be one of the best of his poetical achievements. The following extracts will give an idea of his state of mind at that period.

"I am lost in unconquerable desire; there is nothing left but everlasting tears. Let them flow, let them flow unceasingly. But they can never extinguish the fire that burns me. My heart rages; it is torn in pieces, this heart where life and death meet in a horrible combat." "I have lost the universe, I have lost myself, I who until now have been the favourite of the gods; they have put me to the question, they offered me Pandora, rich in treasure and still richer in perilous seductions; they made me drunken with the kisses of her mouth, which gave me its sweets; they have torn me from her arms, and have struck me with death."

Goethe concealed his elegy for some time, guarding it as something sacred, but eventually handed it over to Eckermann. Poetic creation soothed his mind only for a time. His nature demanded some more efficacious consolation. A few weeks after the separation he began to complain bitterly of the absence of the Countess Julie von Egloffstein, whom he wanted very much. "She cannot know what she is keeping from me and what she makes me lose, nor can she know how I love her and how she engrosses my mind." He derived a little comfort from the visits of Madame Szymanowska, whom he admired "not only as a great artist, but as a pretty woman" (Eckermann, Nov. 3, 1823). "I am deeply grateful to this charming woman," he said to the chancellor, "for her beauty, her sweetness, and her art have soothed my passionate heart" (Bode, p. 151). He also renewed his relations with Marianne Jung, the retired actress and dancer. "When Goethe had to turn his thoughts from Ulrique, the image of the pretty owner of Gerbermühle again occupied his mind. A visit to her, and intimate correspondence with her, restored peace to his heart so greedy of love" (Bielschowsky, vol. ii, p. 487).

His devotion to Ulrique was Goethe's last acute attack of love; but until the end of his days he felt the need of being surrounded by pretty women. As director of the theatre, he came in contact with many young women who wished engagements. He confessed to Eckermann that he required much strength of mind to resist feminine charms which tempted him to be unjustly favourable to the prettiest of those who sought employment. "If I allowed myself to fall into an intrigue of gallantry, I would become like a demagnetised needle as soon as the girl found a real lover" (Eckermann, March 22, 1825).

His daughter-in-law's sister has related that Goethe liked to have young girls in his study whilst he was at work. They had to sit quietly, neither working nor talking, often a difficult task for them (Bode, p. 155).

Even on the last day of his life, whilst in delirium, he cried out, "What a pretty woman's head with black curls on a black ground" (Lewes, vol. ii, p. 372). After uttering several other more or less incoherent phrases, he drew his last breath.

The facts which I described in the chapter of this book dealing with old age have made clear how long sexuality persists in men. As the testes resist atrophy better than other organs, and even in extreme old age still form active spermatozoa, it is natural that their condition should be reflected on the organism generally, and that feelings of love should still be excited. If by some accident

Goethe had become a eunuch early in life, he would have been a different being. The moralists who have been shocked by his amorous intrigues would have been satisfied, but the world would have lost a great poet. Moreover, Goethe is no exceptional case amongst writers. The temperament of Victor Hugo and his devotion to women up to the end of his days are well known. More recently, after the death of Ibsen, a profound sensation was made by the revelation of his love for Mademoiselle Bardach, who inspired his genius during the last period of his life.

Not only poetic creation but other forms of genius are intimately associated with the sexual function. The philosopher Schopenhauer, who was no ascetic, wrote as follows, at the age of twenty-five, when he was in full creative activity, " In the days and at the hours when the voluptuous instinct is strongest, when it is a burning covetousness, it is then that the greatest forces of the mind and the greatest stores of knowledge are ready for the most intense activity." "At such moments life is truly at its strongest and most active, for its two poles are then operating most actively; and this is plain in the man of the highest intelligence. In these hours one sees more than in years of passivity " (quoted in Moebius' *Schopenhauer*, p. 55). " This means that in Schopenhauer intellectual creation was linked with erotic excitement " (*ibid.*, p. 57).

It was facts of such a nature that led Brown-Séquard to his idea of strengthening cerebral activity by injections of the substance of testes. To obtain the same effect, he prescribed another means, the value of which was proved in the case of two individuals aged from forty-five to fifty years, the observations being continued over several years. " By my advice," he said, " when these had to perform any great physical or intellectual work, they got themselves into a condition of sexual excitement." " The testes being in this way thrown into functional activity, there was soon produced the desired increase in the power of the nerve centres."[1]

Although I insist on the existence of a close relation between intellectual activity and the sexual function, I do not mean to assert that there have not existed exceptions to the rule.

Now that I have described certain important factors in the genius of Goethe, I shall pass on to a study of his state of mind in the last period of his life, the splendour and harmony of which have been so often admired.

[1] *Comptes rendus de la Société de Biologie*, 1889, p. 420.

III

GOETHE'S OLD AGE

Old age of Goethe—Physical and intellectual vigour of the old man—Optimistic conception of life—Happiness in life in his last period

DRINKERS of wine may take the case of Goethe as an argument against temperance. Although he was not healthy in his youth, his large consumption of wine did not prevent him from enjoying an old age full of force and intellectual work. Eckermann, who was his intimate and constant companion in the last ten years of his life, was never weary of expressing his surprise and delight at the physical and moral vigour of the distinguished old man. He found Goethe on his return to Jena, at the age of seventy-four, in a condition "very pleasant to see; he was in good health and robust, so that he could walk for hours" (Sept. 15, 1823). His eyes were "brilliant and clear and his whole expression was that of joy, vigour and youth" (Oct. 29). In walks with Eckermann, Goethe forced the pace and showed strength which filled his companion with delight (March, 1824). His voice was full of character and of force (March 30, 1824), and every word showed his vitality (July 9, 1827).

In a conversation that Eckermann had with Goethe when the latter was seventy-nine years old "the sound of his voice and the fire in his eyes were of such strength as would have been normal in the full flush of youth" (Mar. 11, 1828). Such characters were preserved until the end of the life of the great man, and a few months before his death Eckermann jotted in his book that he saw him every day in full vigour and freshness, looking as if his health might be prolonged indefinitely (Dec. 21, 1831). In the beginning of the following spring, Goethe caught a feverish cold, possibly pneumonic, and died, probably from weakness of the heart. His illness lasted a week. If he had not been a drinker of wine he would have been able to withstand this attack and to live still longer.

The intellectual vigour of Goethe was even greater and more remarkable than his physical strength. His interests were extremely wide, and his thirst for knowledge was never appeased. Once, when he was absorbed by the interest of hearing d'Alton describe in detail the skeleton of rodents, Eckermann states his surprise that a man not far short of eighty years old "did not give up seeking for and gaining knowledge." But in these matters he never lost his interest. He wished always to go further and further, always to learn, so showing himself to be a man of eternal and undying youth (April 16, 1825). Goethe's aptitude for understanding and his memory were most unusual. When he was more than eighty, he surprised those who heard him "by the incessant flow of his ideas and by his extraordinary fertility in invention" (Oct. 7, 1828).

"The old age of Goethe is the most striking proof of the extreme force of his constitution," said his medical biographer, Dr. Moebius. Works which were written in his last years are for the most part beyond praise, both because of their finished form, and by their wisdom and feeling. What other man of eighty has written anything of the same character? From the physiological point of view I am more surprised at his works when he was old than at those of his youthful activity " (Moebius, *Goethe,* i, 200, 201).

Although Goethe's character, which was fiery and intense in his youth, became much more calm with age, there still came to him moments when he was carried away. He had certain eccentricities of an old man, and in particular was often very despotic, and this trait has been the occasion of many stories. His temper, however, became much more certain in his old age, and his general conceptions much more optimistic. Apart from certain short crises, he was happy in his life. In 1828, he settled down at Dornburg and there passed a tranquil existence. " I stay out of doors nearly all day and engage in private conversations with the tendrils of the vine which communicate their excellent ideas to me, ideas about which I shall have marvellous things to tell you "—he wrote to Eckermann on June 15, 1828—" I am composing verses which are quite good, and I hope that it will be given to me to live long in this condition. I am quite contented," he said to his collaborator, " at the beginning of spring, when I see the first green leaves, I am pleased to watch how, from week to week, one leaf after another appears on the stem. I am delighted in May, when I see a flower-bud; I feel really happy, when in June the rose offers to me its splendour and its perfume " (Eckermann, April 27, 1825). His delight in life at this epoch is also revealed in many letters. " I wish to whisper this in your ear," he wrote to Zelter on April 29, 1830. " I am delighted to find that even at my great age, ideas come to me the pursuit and development of which would require a second life."

His conception of life had changed enormously since the epoch of *Werther.* Goethe himself said: " When one is old, one thinks many things about this world quite different from when one was young " (Eckermann, Dec.,

1829). The youthful sensitiveness which had brought him so much suffering was notably dulled. Eckermann was astonished at the way he accepted wounds to his pride. It happened that his design for the new theatre at Weimar was abandoned while it was being constructed, and replaced by another not his own work. Eckermann was much disturbed by this, and went to see Goethe in a state of apprehension. "I was afraid," he said, "that so unexpected a step would profoundly wound Goethe. Well, there was nothing of the sort; I found him in the best of tempers, quite calm, absolutely above all feelings in the matter." When he had reached his eighty-fourth year, Goethe had no weariness of life. In his last illness, he showed not the smallest desire to die. He expected to get better, and thought that the approach of summer would restore his strength. The desire to live was strong in him. None the less, he recognised that his cycle of life was finished, and although he had no weariness of life, he felt a kind of satisfaction that life was over. "When, like me, a man has lived eighty years," he said, "he has hardly the right to live, but ought to be ready every day to die, and to think of putting his house in order" (Eckermann, May 15, 1831). None the less, he continued his work, in particular revising the last two chapters of the second part of *Faust*. When he had finished them, Goethe was extremely pleased. "I can consider," he said, "any days which come to me yet as a real gift, as it is a matter of no moment if I write anything more or what such work should be" (Eckermann, June 1, 1831).

Goethe gave Faust one hundred years of life, and it is probable that he thought of that period as his own span. Although he did not reach it, he approached it, after having lived a most active life, full of most valuable lessons for posterity.

IV

GOETHE AND "FAUST"

Faust the biography of Goethe--The three monologues in the first Part—Faust's pessimism—The brain-fatigue which finds a remedy in love—The romance with Marguerite and its unhappy ending

"GOETHE was Faust, Faust Goethe," said the biographer of the great poet (Bielschowsky, vol. ii, p. 645). Most people admit that in *Faust* Goethe gave his autobiography on a more detailed scale than in *Werther*. Why then should I follow my analysis of Goethe himself, which was based on exact facts, with an analysis of Faust? I do so because in addition to the biographical details in *Faust*, there are many ideas which illuminate the poet's conception of life. Goethe's life explains *Faust*, and *Faust* explains the soul of its author. And I am convinced that an accurate study of so great a man is of high importance in the investigation of human nature.

The two Parts of *Faust* correspond with two distinct periods in Goethe's life. In the first Part, Faust was pessimistic, in the second optimistic. Although many of the high problems that occupy humanity are raised and discussed in *Faust*, love is the centre on which the drama turns.

In the first Part, conceived and for the most part written

during his youth, the chief theme is the love of a young man for a pretty and attractive girl towards whom the hero acts in a fashion opposed to conventional morality. As in most of his principal works, Goethe has made an episode in his own life the basis of *Faust.* It is the well-known story of Frederique, the daughter of a clergyman, for whom the brilliant young author conceived a violent passion and who returned his affection with a deeper and more enduring feeling. Goethe was alarmed at the possibility of definitely settling his future, and deserted the poor victim of love in an unfortunate state. Later on, he confessed to the Baroness von Stein that he had abandoned Frederique at a time when his desertion was likely to cause the death of the poor girl. "I had wounded to the quick," he wrote (Bielschowsky, vol. i, p. 135), "the best heart in the world, and I had to repent of it long and almost unendurably." As an atonement, he made Frederique the heroine of "Goetz" and of "Clavigo," but not thinking these worthy of her, he immortalised her as the Marguerite of *Faust.*

A learned doctor, skilled in all human knowledge, but who had found no satisfaction in his studies, found consolation in the beauty and charm of a young girl with whom he fell passionately in love. It will be interesting to trace the psychological process which induced him to leave the scene of his scientific studies for the streets and resorts where he found Marguerite.

Although Faust was represented as an old man, who had had time enough to absorb all human learning, his image bears the stamp of green youth. "Discontented with all his knowledge, he wished to know the secret entrails of the world, to be a witness of the centre of all activity, to unveil the principle of life."[1] These are the demands of a young

[1] The word *Samen* of the original is the expression of the alchemists for the "principle of life."

man seeking to resolve the most intricate problems at one stroke. The speech in question dates from the period of *Werther*, when Goethe was twenty-five years old, and for that reason leaves no very serious impression.[1] The second monologue, which ends with the attempt to take poison, is later, and is absent in the edition of 1790 (Fragment). It was revised when Goethe had reached his fiftieth year, and displays a riper maturity. Although lacking exactness, it depicts in an interesting fashion the miseries of life.

> Some alien substance more and more is cleaving
> To all the mind conceives of grand and fair;
> When this world's Good is won by our achieving,
> The Better, then, is named a cheat and snare.
> The fine emotions, whence our lives we mould,
> Lie in the earthly tumult dumb and cold.
> If hopeful Fancy once, in daring flight,
> Her longings to the Infinite expanded,
> Yet now a narrow space contents her quite,
> Since Time's wild wave so many a fortune stranded.
> Care at the bottom of the heart is lurking;
> Her secret pangs in silence working,
> She, restless, rocks herself, disturbing joy and rest;
> In newer masks her face is ever drest,
> By turns as house and land, as wife and child, presented,—
> As water, fire, as poison, steel;
> We dread the blows we never feel,
> And what we never lose is yet by us lamented.

Fear of the evils which lie in wait for us and against which we can make no provision render life insupportable. Faust's frame of mind as described in these lines recalls Schopenhauer, who was always afraid of something; fear, sometimes of thieves, sometimes of diseases, tormented

---

[1] Erich Schmidt, Goethe's *Faust in ursprünglicher Gestalt*, 6th edit., Weimar, 1905, p. 1.
[2] *Faust*, Bayard Taylor's translation. London: Warne & Co., pp. 20-21.

him. He would never go to a barber's to be shaved, and always carried his own drinking cup with him.

"Is it not better to end such a life, and to kill oneself, even if it mean annihilation?" asked Faust. He took up the poisoned goblet and put it to his lips, but, arrested by singing and the sound of bells outside, he refrained, and life laid hold of him. Not religious faith, however, but memories of childhood, "the happy sports of youth and the gay festivals of spring" were the agencies that recalled Faust to the earth. He went out of doors, mingled with the crowd, tried to amuse himself amongst men, and savoured the beauty of the new-born spring, but all these could not make him forget the evil of life. He met his pupil, talked with him, and again displayed his pessimism.

> O happy he, who still renews
> The hope, from Error's deeps to rise for ever!
> That which one does not know, one needs to use;
> And what one knows, one uses never.[1]

Then follows the celebrated monologue of Faust over which so many commentators have lost their heads and wasted oceans of ink.

> Two souls, alas! reside within my breast,
> And each withdraws from, and repels, its brother.
> One with tenacious organs holds in love
> And clinging lust the world in its embraces;
> The other strongly sweeps, this dust above,
> Into the high ancestral spaces.[2]

On this passage has been built up a whole theory of "double natures" with which has been incorporated the dualism of Manicheism, the two natures of Christ and what not besides.[3]

---

[1] *Op. cit.*, p. 32.
[2] *Op. cit.*, pp. 33, 34.
[3] Details of this will be found in Kuno Fischer's *Goethe's Faust*, pp. 328–330.

There exists in literature no better expression of human disharmony than this monologue " of the two souls." It portrays the unbalanced condition so frequent in youth and is a valuable indication of the real youth of Faust.

On his return to his study, Faust again revealed his pessimism.

> But ah! I feel, though will thereto be stronger,
> Contentment flows from out my breast no longer.
> Why must the stream so soon run dry and fail us,
> And burning thirst again assail us?
> Therein I've borne so much probation! [1]

It is at this point that Faust addresses the Spirit " that denies " and that is called " sin " and " evil." This spirit invokes before his eyes "the fairest images of dreams," that is to say, a woman's body in its beautiful nudity. Faust declares himself

> Too old to play with passion,
> Too young to be without desire. [2]

Pursued by desire

> .... when night descends, how anxiously
> Upon my couch of sleep I lay me.
> There, also, comes no rest to me;
> But some wild dream is sent to fray me. [3]

So that

> Death is desired, and Life a thing unblest.
> O fortunate, for whom, when victory glances,
> The bloody laurels on the brow he bindeth!
> Whom, after rapid, maddening dances,
> In clasping maiden-arms he findeth! [4]

Faust thus reached the ecstasy of passion. Soon afterwards in the Witches' kitchen, he saw in a mirror a " heavenly form " and cried:—

> O lend me, Love, the swiftest of thy pinions,
> And bear me to her beauteous field.

[1] *Op. cit.*, p. 36. [2] *Op. cit.*, p. 45
[3] *Op. cit.*, p. 46. [4] *Op. cit.*, p. 46.

> A woman's form, in beauty shining!
> Can woman, then, so lovely be?
> And must I find her body, there reclining;
> Of all the heavens, the bright epitome?
> Can Earth with such a thing be mated?[1]

Discontent with life, sense of the insufficiency of human knowledge and the most gloomy pessimism lead to the passion of love which, eventually, after many devious paths, throws Faust into the arms of Marguerite. The story is one of the world's great romances and everyone knows it. Faust all unconsciously was following the prescription of Brown-Séquard. Brain-fatigue had made the continuation of the study which caused it impossible. The condition is plainly stated in the following lines:—

> The thread of Thought at last is broken,
> And knowledge brings disgust unspoken.
> Let us the sensual deeps explore.[2]

The brain has refused to work, and blind instinct, in the guise of dreams, whispers that there is in the organism something that can restore the intellectual forces. This something, however, is what is called sin, and much courage is needed to plunge into it. Without this evil, life cannot last. Faust has to choose between love and death, and chooses love.

The end of the romance of Goethe and Frederique was bad, and that of Faust and Marguerite was still worse. The poet painted it in the most sombre colours. Marguerite killed her child, poisoned her mother, became crazy, and was beheaded. Faust's cup of misery was filled to the brim; he blamed his evil genius, he made desperate efforts to save the poor woman, and cried "O that I had never been born."

To sum up: in the first Part, Faust is a young, learned man who expects too much from science and life, and whose

[1] *Op. cit.*, p. 71. [2] *Op. cit.*, p. 51.

genius requires extra-conjugal love as a stimulant; he is unbalanced and inevitably pessimistic. It is not surprising that his life goes badly, and that his conduct leaves him much to repent of. But although, at first, a vague general discontent nearly drives him to suicide, later on the terrible evil which he had wrought on a poor creature he loved passionately did no more than plunge him into misery that was bitter but far from mortal. His mind had developed far in the direction of optimism. The crisis through which he passed, serious as it was, ended by his return to a life of great activity and enterprise.

V

THE OLD AGE OF FAUST

The second Part of Faust is in the main a description of senile love—Amorous passion of the old man—Humble attitude of the old Faust—Platonic love for Helena—The old Faust's conception of life—His optimism—The general idea of the play

THE first Part of *Faust* was acclaimed by the world almost as soon as it appeared, but the second Part met a very cold reception. Everyone knows and reads the first Part; the second Part has few readers, and these chiefly poets and dramatists. No doubt it has more effect on the stage than when it is read, but this is due to subsidiary features in which it resembles a fine ballet. There is general agreement that the real meaning of the second Part is obscure, complex and difficult to interpret. Many literary critics have racked their brains in the effort to discover the author's central idea. When Eckermann, who persuaded Goethe to revise and finish the second Part, asked what was the meaning of some of the scenes in it, Goethe evaded the question and played the sphinx. Thus, with regard to the famous " mothers " Goethe answered, with a mysterious air :—" You have the manuscript: study it, and see what you can make of it " (January 10, 1830). G. H. Lewes, although one of Goethe's most resolute admirers, admitted the impossibility of grasping the sense of the second Part. The Wanderjahre and the second Part of *Faust* were arsenals of symbols, and it pleased the old poet to see acute critics labouring to interpret them whilst he was silent and refused to help them. Lewes thought that Goethe, so far from showing the smallest wish to clear up their difficulties, took a pleasure in giving them new problems to puzzle over. Lewes himself thought that the second Part was poor in idea and execution, and admitted that he had failed after repeatedly trying to get a conception of it that would reveal its beauties. In writing about it, he contented himself with giving a summary of it. Now this second Part, although its general lines had been laid down for long, was actually written during several years in the last period of the poet's life. The fact that it was composed out of the regular sequence of the Acts and Scenes gives us an important clue. The third Act and then the second Part of the fifth Act were put on paper first. Next followed the first Act and part of the second; the classical Walpurgis night was written in 1830, the fourth Act in 1831, and last of all the beginning of the fifth Act.

As the second Part of *Faust* is a crowded motley, containing many subjects, obviously of minor importance, such as the volcanic theory of the earth and the disquisition on paper-money, the key-note may be found in the portions which were first composed. Now Act III. contains the story of Helena, and the second part of Act V. Faust's activity for the general welfare.

Setting out from the conception that the works of Goethe reflect the acts and incidents of his own life, I shall try to explain on that basis the meaning of the most obscure of his writings.

I have already stated that love was the stimulus of

Goethe's activity in youth and age; it is the scarlet thread running through his history. There was no difficulty in his using his love for Frederique as material for a play; that a young man should love a young girl was natural enough. The story of an old man enamoured of a young beauty was quite another matter. It was said that one of the reasons that prevented his marriage with Ulrique de Lewetzow was the fear of ridicule (Lewes, *op. cit.*, ii, p. 345), a fear that plays a large part in human affairs. It is easy to understand that the old poet was in a difficulty when he came to write of senile love. Faust's love for Helena was not that of a supposed old man who became young by doffing his beard and changing his cloak, but of a real old man whom no mystery nor magic was to make young again. And yet old Faust's love was a true passion, and Goethe has written no finer lines than those describing it.

When the second Part begins, Faust has passed through the terrible crisis of the first Part. Wearied and restless, he seeks a new mode of life.

> Life's pulses now with fresher force awaken
> To greet the mild ethereal twilight o'er me;
> This night, thou, Earth! hast also stood unshaken,
> And now thou breathest, new-refreshed before me,
> And now beginnest, all thy gladness granting,
> A vigorous resolution to restore me,
> To seek that higher life for which I'm panting.[1]

The invoked image of the most beautiful woman in the history of the world transforms Faust's desire of love into an overwhelming passion.

> Have I still eyes? Deep in my being springs
> The fount of Beauty, in a torrent pouring!
> A heavenly gain my path of terror brings.
> The world was void, and shut to my exploring,—

[1] *Op. cit.*, p. 151.

THE OLD AGE OF FAUST

> And, since my priesthood, how hath it been graced!
> Enduring 'tis, desirable, firm-based.
> And let my breath of being blow to waste,
> If I for thee unlearn my sacred duty!
> The form, that long erewhile my fancy captured,
> That from the magic mirror so enraptured,
> Was but a frothy phantom of such beauty!
> 'Tis Thou, to whom the stir of all my forces,
> The essence of my passion's courses,—
> Love, fancy, worship, madness,—here I render.[1]

In the throes of this passion, Faust is tortured by jealousy when he sees the lovely woman clinging to and kissing a young man. He desires her at all costs.

> Am I nothing here? To stead me,
> Is not this key still shining in my hand?
> Through realms of terror, wastes and waves it led me,
> Through solitudes, to where I firmly stand,
> Here foothold is! Realities here centre!
> The strife with spirits here the mind may venture,
> And on its grand, its double lordship enter!
> How far she was, and nearer, how divine!
> I'll rescue her and make her doubly mine.
> Ye Mothers! Mothers! Crown this wild endeavour!
> Who knows her once must hold her, and for ever.[2]

The disappearance of the beautiful woman so moved Faust that he fainted and fell into a prolonged sleep. As soon as he recovered consciousness he asked: "Where is she?" and set out to seek for her. When he learned that Chiron had already carried off Helena on his back Faust cried out:—

> Her didst thou bear?
> *Chiron:* This back she pressed.
> *Faust:* Was I not wild enough, before;
> And now such seat, to make me blest!
> O, I scarcely dare
> To trust my senses!—tell me more!
> She is my only aspiration!
> Whence didst thou bear her—to what shore?[3]

[1] *Op. cit.*, p. 203.   [2] *Op. cit.* p. 205.   [3] *Op. cit.*, p. 230.

> Thou saw'st her once; *to-day* I saw her beam,
> The dream of Beauty, beautiful as Dream!
> My soul, my being, now is bound and chained;
> I cannot live, unless she be attained.[1]

Chiron found this attitude of passionate emotion so strange that he advised Faust to take care of his health.

After many wanderings and difficulties Faust again met the woman he coveted and spoke to her as follows:—

> What else remains, but that I give to thee
> Myself, and all I vainly fancied mine?
> Let me, before thy feet, in fealty true,
> Thee now acknowledge, Lady, whose approach
> Won thee at once possession and the throne![2]

This language, so very different from what the same man had formerly addressed to Marguerite, is much more like that of an old lover to a young beauty whom he admires. When Helena invited Faust to sit on the throne beside her, he replied:—

> First, kneeling, let the dedication be
> Accepted, lofty Lady! Let me kiss
> The gracious hand that lifts me to thy side.
> Confirm me as co-regent of thy realm,
> Whose borders are unknown, and win for thee
> Guard, slave and worshipper, and all in one![3]

The old man in the throes of a passion so great that he was wholly absorbed by it did not dare to address the beloved woman except in the most humble terms.

Helena made no declaration of love, but was complacent to him, and when Faust suggested: "Now let our throne become a bower unblighted," Helena agreed to follow him to a secluded and green bower. There they remained alone for some time, cared for by an old servant.

The result of this union was not a child like that to which Marguerite gave birth and afterwards killed. It was a

---

[1] *Op. cit.*, p. 231.   [2] *Op. cit.*, p. 284.   [3] *Op. cit.*, p. 287.

strange and peculiar being; a boy who immediately after his birth began to leap about and to alarm his parents by the activity of his movements.

Although Goethe preserved an obstinate silence when he was asked to explain many of the scenes in the second Part, he had no hesitation in explaining the significance of this astonishing child. "The child was not a human being but an allegory, in which was personified poetry, which is not bound to any time, to any place, or to any person" (Eckermann, December 20, 1829). Struck by the tragic fate of Byron, Goethe made the son of Faust and Helena a symbol of the English poet.

Literary critics, setting out from the categorical explanation of Goethe himself, have declared that the union of Faust and Helena was meant to denote the alliance of romanticism and classicism, a marriage from which was born modern poetry, personified in its highest representative, Byron. This, however, cannot be the idea of Goethe, who himself was far from an enthusiast about classicism and romanticism. "What," he said, "is all this noise about the classic and the romantic? The essential thing is that a piece of work should be wholly good and serious; then it will also be classic" (Eckermann, October 17, 1828). It is much more probable that Goethe intended poetry to spring from the relations between the old Faust and his adorable companion, relations of a kind to be included in so-called platonic love. Such love inspires the creation of perfect work even in an old poet, when he is stimulated by a beautiful woman.

When Faust and Helena emerged from the grotto with their son, Helena said:—

>   *Helena:* Love, in human wise to bless us,
>   In a noble pair must be;

> But divinely to possess us,
> It must form a precious Three.

Faust: All we seek has therefore found us;
I am thine and thou art mine!
So we stand as love hath bound us;
Other fortune we resign.[1]

After the death of her son, Helena abandoned Faust, leaving him her garments:—

Helena: Also in me, alas! an old word proves its truth,
That Bliss and Beauty ne'er enduringly unite.
Torn is the link of Life, no less than that of Love;
So, both lamenting, painfully I say: Farewell!
And cast myself again,—once only,—in thine arms.[2]

After this crisis the old Faust sought to console himself in the bosom of nature, just as after the terrible catastrophe with Marguerite the contemplation of nature had given him the strength to live. On this occasion he reached the summit of a high mountain from which he watched the changing vapours of a cloud which seemed to him to assume the form of female beauty. But Faust was old, and now saw only memories of love. He cried out:—

> Yes! mine eyes not err!—
> On sun-illumined pillows beauteously reclined,
> Colossal, truly, but a godlike woman-form,
> I see! The like of Juno, Leda, Helena,
> Majestically lovely, floats before my sight!
> Ah! now 'tis broken! Towering broad and formlessly,
> It rests along the east like distant icy hills,
> And shapes the grand significance of fleeting days.
> Yet still there clings a light and delicate band of mist
> Around my breast and brow, caressing, cheering me.
> Now light, delaying, it soars and higher soars,
> And folds together.—Cheats me an ecstatic form,
> As early-youthful, long-foregone and highest bliss?
> The first glad treasures of my deepest heart break forth;
> Aurora's love, so light of pinion, is its type,
> The swiftly-felt, the first, scarce-comprehended glance,
> Outshining every treasure, when retained and held.

[1] *Op. cit.*, p 298.   *Op. cit.*, p. 305.

> Like Spiritual Beauty mounts the gracious Form,
> Dissolving not, but lifts itself through ether far,
> And from my inner being bears the best away.[1]

This state of mind resembles Goethe's condition after the rupture with Ulrique.

Love and poetry alike were over for him. None the less his craving for the higher life was not yet weakened. The desire to live was still very strong in the old Faust. But now he no longer as in the days of his youth dreamed of an ideal which could not be attained. When Mephistopheles asked him ironically:—

> Then might one guess whereunto thou hast striven?
> Boldly-sublime it was, I'm sure.
> Since nearer to the moon thy flight was driven,
> Would now thy mania that realm secure?
>
> *Faust:* Not so! This sphere of earthly soil
> Still gives us room for lofty doing.
> Astounding plans e'en now are brewing:
> I feel new strength for bolder toil.[2]

Such optimistic language, extraordinarily different from Faust's lamentations in the first Part, becomes still more marked. When he was approaching his centenary he made the following profession of faith:—

> I only through the world have flown:
> Each appetite I seized as by the hair;
> What not sufficed me, forth I let it fare,
> And what escaped me, I let go.
> I've only craved, accomplished my delight,
> Then wished a second time, and thus with might
> Stormed through my life: at first 'twas grand, completely,
> But now it moves most wisely and discreetly.
> The sphere of Earth is known enough to me;
> The view beyond is barred immutably:
> A fool, who there his blinking eyes directeth,
> And o'er his clouds of peers a place expecteth!
> Firm let him stand, and look around him well!
> This World means something to the Capable.
> Why needs he through Eternity to wend?
> He here acquires what he can appreheand.[3]

[1] *Op. cit.*, p. 309.   [2] *Op. cit.*, p. 313.   [3] *Op. cit.*, p. 351.

When he had reached the maturity of his wisdom, Faust organised drainage works, the object of which was to increase the area of land that could be utilised:—

> To many millions let me furnish soil,
> Though not secure, yet free to active toil;
> Green, fertile fields.
> A land like Paradise here, round about.
> Yes! to this thought I hold with firm persistence;
> The last result of wisdom stamps it true:
> He only earns his freedom and existence,
> Who daily conquers them anew.
> Thus here, by dangers girt, shall glide away
> Of childhood, manhood, age, the vigorous day:
> And such a throng I fain would see,
> Stand on free soil among a people free!
> Then dared I hail the Moment fleeing:
> " Ah, still delay—thou art so fair! "
> The traces cannot, of mine earthly being,
> In æons perish,—they are there!—
> In proud fore-feeling of such lofty bliss,
> I now enjoy the highest Moment,—this! [1]

These were the last words of the wise centenarian. It has been said that they contain the quintessence of Goethe's moral philosophy, and that they preach the sacrifice of the individual for the benefit of society. Lewes, for instance, takes this view, holding that Faust was the exposition of a man who had conquered the vanity of individual aspirations and joys, and had come to the knowledge of the great truth that man must live for man, and can find lasting happiness only in work for the benefit of humanity. For my own part, it seems to me that according to Goethe's *Faust* man must dedicate a large part of his life to the complete development of his own individuality, and that it is only in the second half of his life, when he has grown wise by experience and feels satisfied as an individual, that he should use his activity for the good of

[1] *Op. cit.*, pp. 354-355.

mankind. It was no part either of the ideas of Goethe or of the nature of his work to preach the sacrifice of individuality.

Goethe was thus absorbed in *Faust* by the problem of the conflict between certain actions and guiding principles. The misdeeds of the hero in the first Part of his life had to be redeemed. He said to Eckermann that "the key to the salvation of Faust was to be found in the Angels' Chorus":—

> The noble spirit now is free,
> And saved from evil scheming:
> Whoe'er aspires unweariedly
> Is not beyond redeeming.[1]

However, that of which he did not speak, and which none the less was most important in Faust and in Goethe himself, is the action of love as a stimulant to artistic creation, and it was probably to this that he referred at the end of his tragedy. The mystical chorus sent up prayers in a religious and erotic ecstasy, and their mysterious song is:—

> The Indescribable,
> Here it is done;
> The Woman-Soul leadeth us
> Upward and on![2]

Although these verses have been interpreted as love which sacrifices or even love which leads to the grace of God (Bode, p. 149), it is much more probable that it is love for feminine beauty, a love which makes possible the execution of wonderful things. Such an interpretation agrees with the fact that the verses are spoken by a *mystic* choir which speaks of the *indescribable* (*das Unbeschreibliche*) in which we must see the amorous passion of the old man. In such an interpretation the whole of *Faust* (and especially the second Part) is an eloquent pleading

[1] *Op. cit.*, p. 365.   [2] *Op. cit.*, p. 370.

for the importance of love in the higher activity of man, in accordance with the law of human nature, which is a much better justification of Goethe's conduct than all the arguments of his interpreters and admirers.

I do not agree with the common idea that the two Parts of *Faust* are two distinct works, but regard them as complementary. In the first Part we see the young pessimist, full of ardour and of desires, ready to make an end of his days and stopping at nothing to satisfy his thirst for love. In the second Part we have a mature old man still loving women, but in a different way, a man who is wise and optimistic, and who, having satiated the wants of his individual life, dedicates the rest of his days to mankind, and who, having reached a century, dies extremely happy, in fact almost exhibiting the instinct of natural death.

PART IX

SCIENCE AND MORALITY

I

UTILITARIAN AND INTUITIVE MORALITY

Difficulty of the problem of morality—Vivisection and antivivisection—Enquiry into the possibility of rational morality—Utilitarian and intuitive theories of morality—Insufficiency of these

In the course of this book I have from time to time approached subjects closely related with the problem of morality. For instance, in considering the prolongation of human life, it was necessary to show that extension of longevity far beyond the reproductive period of man in no way is opposed to the principles of the highest morality, although there exist races who find the sacrifice of old people in harmony with their conception of morality.

Experimental biology, which lies at the root of most of the doctrines exposed in this work, depends on vivisection of animals. There are, however, very many persons who regard it as immoral to operate on living animals when it is not for the direct benefit of these. The attempts which have been made in France and Germany to prevent or to limit vivisection in laboratories have not succeeded, but in England there is a severe law controlling operations on animals and submitting them to oppressive regulations to which many of the scientific men in the country are opposed.

The question of experiments upon human beings is still

more delicate. Just as formerly the examination of a human corpse could be made only in secret, so at the present time, if the slightest experiment is to be made upon a human being, it can be only by devious ways. People who are hardly shocked at all at the numberless accidents caused by automobiles and other means of transit, or in field sports, make the strongest protest against any proposal to try some new method of treatment upon a human being.

A large number of people, amongst them even men of science, regard as immoral any attempt to prevent the spread of venereal diseases. Recently, in connection with the investigations into the action of mercurial ointment as a means of preventing syphilis, the members of the Faculty of Medicine in France made a public protest, declaring that it would be "immoral to let people think that they could indulge in sexual vice without danger," and that it was "wrong to give to the public a means of protection in debauch."[1] None the less, other men of science, equally serious, were convinced that they were performing an absolutely moral work in attempting to find a prophylactic against syphilis which would preserve many people, including children and other innocent persons who, if no preventive measures existed, would suffer from the terrible disease.

Such examples show the reader what confusion exists in the problem of morality. Although at every moment, in every act of human conduct, the precepts of morality must be reckoned with, even the most authoritative persons are far from agreeing as to what rules to follow. About a year ago in a Parisian journal[2] an enquiry into the subject

[1] *V. Tribune médicale*, 1906, p. 449.
[2] *La Revue*, Nov. 15th and Dec. 1st.

of rational morality was directed to distinguished authors. The object was to discover if, at the present time, moral conduct could be based not on religious dogma, which binds only those who believe in it, but on rational principles. The answers were most contradictory. Some denied the possibility of rational morality, others admitted it, but in very different fashions. Whilst one philosopher, M. Boutroux, held that "morality must be founded on reason and could have no other foundation," a poet, M. Sully-Prudhomme, turned to feeling and conscience as the basis of morality. According to him, " in the teaching of morality, it is the heart and not the mind which is at once master and pupil." In the contradictions which I mentioned in the beginning of this chapter, these two views appear. When antivivisectionists are protesting against experiments on animals, they are inspired by sympathy for poor creatures which cannot defend themselves. Guided by conscience, they think immoral any suffering inflicted upon a living being for the benefit of another being, whether human or animal. I know distinguished physiologists who have determined to limit their experiments to animals with little sensibility, such as frogs. The great majority of scientific men, however, would have no scruple in opening bodies and subjecting their victims to severe suffering in the hope of clearing up some scientific problem which sooner or later would increase the happiness of human beings and animals. If vivisection had not been performed, or if it had been restricted, the great laws of infectious diseases would not have been discovered, nor would the discovery of many valuable remedies have been made. To justify investigation, men of science set out from the utilitarian theory of morality, which approves everything that is useful to the human race. The antivivisectionists, on the other hand, rely on the intuitive theory, according to which conduct is controlled by the spontaneous activity of our conscience.

In the case which I have selected the problem is easy to solve. It is plain that vivisection is inevitable in the experimental investigation of vital processes, as it is the only means by whch serious progress can be made. None the less, very many people cannot accept this necessity, because of the intensity of their love for animals.

In the question of the prevention of syphilis, the moral problem is still more easy to settle. Whilst in the case of vivisection a real suffering may be inflicted upon animals, in preventive measures against syphilis, the evil is more or less intricate and very problematic. The certainty of safety from this disease might render extra-conjugal relations more frequent, but if we compare the evil which might come from that with the immense benefit gained in preventing so many innocent persons from becoming diseased, it is easy to see to which side the scale dips. The indignation of those who protest against the discovery of preventive measures can never either arrest the zeal of the investigators or hinder the use of the measures. This example again shows that reasoning is necessary in the solution of most moral questions.

However, the problems which arise in actual life are often very much more complicated than the two cases I have taken as an introduction. It is easy to prove the high utility of the work of vivisectors and of those who are seeking means of preventing syphilis, whilst their adversaries have nothing to invoke but their feelings. The situation is quite different in many questions which border on morality. The sexual life abounds in extremely difficult problems, in which it is almost impossible to deter-

UTILITARIAN MORALITY

mine what is right. Let me recall the vagaries in the life of Goethe, whose great genius was so often in conflict with the morality of his time. Was he wrong in giving up Frederique and Lili from the fear that a permanent bond would damage his poetic productivity? Then there is the moral question of the marriage of men affected with syphilis, or other diseases which might influence the offspring. The problems of the continence of young people before marriage, of prostitution and of means of preventing conception are without doubt questions of great importance, the solution of which is extremely difficult from the point of view of morality. Differences of opinion are revealed in nearly everything relating to punishment. The question of the death penalty is much in dispute and requires numerous investigations of different kinds. Statistics have been collected to give information as to the utility or inutility of the death penalty. According to some results, capital punishment does not diminish the number of crimes, whilst according to others it has a real preventive effect. Punishments less violent than death, and particularly the punishments of children, are equally troublesome, and schoolmasters have difficulty in finding a solution.

The utilitarian theory of morality often finds it impossible to prove the advantage of the conduct it prescribes, and this the more because in many cases we do not exactly know who is to profit by it. Is the utility of any particular act to be considered so far as it affects relatives, members of the same religion, of the same country, or of the same race, or all humanity?

In face of these difficulties, many moral philosophers have given up the utilitarian theory and declared for an intuitive theory. The basis of morality is to be found in a feeling innate in every man, a sort of social instinct urging him to do good to his neighbour, and which, by the voice of his own conscience, dictates how he ought to act much more precisely than could be done by any comprehension of the utility of his conduct.

It is certainly true that man is an animal living in society because of his need for association with other human beings. But whilst in the animal world the members of societies are actuated by an instinct which is blind and generally very precise, in man we find nothing of the kind. The social instinct appears in him in endless variety. In some of us love of neighbours is extremely highly developed, so that some persons are only happy when sacrificing themselves for the public good. They give all that they have to the poor, and often die for some ideal which is necessarily altruistic. Such examples are rare. Many men, however, profess an affection for some of their kind, devote themselves to their relations, their friends, or their compatriots, and remain practically indifferent to all others. Other individuals, again, have an even narrower sphere of affection, and take advantage of their fellows, either in their own interest or in that of their own family. Still more rare are the really wicked persons who have no love for anyone but themselves and who take pleasure in doing harm to those about them. Notwithstanding this diversity in the development of the social instinct, all men have to live together.

If it were possible to know the inner motives of men, these might be used as a basis for classifying conduct. Those acts might be described as moral which were inspired by neighbourly love, and those as immoral the motive of which was egoism. But it is seldom that the real motives are discovered; they lie deep down in the individual mind, sometimes unknown even to the man himself. We can nearly always harmonise our acts with the dictates of our consciences and find reasons for the harm we inflict upon others. It is only rare natures that possess a conscience so delicate as to be always tormented lest they are not doing good to their neighbours.

In the course of life, men are disposed to attribute bad motives to their opponents. Such an attitude makes criticism easier and panders to the common wish to speak evil of one's neighbours. Notwithstanding the numerous precedents for such an attitude amongst politicians and journalists, it must be discarded from any serious study of morality.

The motives and the conscience are elusive elements of little use in any attempt to value human conduct. We have to fall back on the consequences of action. Now it is easy to show that the social instinct often leads to action which is not good. It frequently happens that men, acting with the highest and best intentions, do much harm. Schopenhauer long ago pointed out that morality based on sentiment is a mere caricature of real morality. Impelled by the altruistic wish to do good, men often lavish unreflecting charity and do harm to others and to themselves. In *Timon of Athens* Shakespeare depicted

> A most incomparable man; breathed, as it were,
> To an untirable and continuate goodness,

and who gave away to the right and the left, creating around him a cloud of parasites. He finally ruined himself and became a hopeless misanthrope. Shakespeare put his verdict in the mouth of Flavius:—

> Undone by goodness. Strange, unusual blood,
> When man's worst sin is, he does too much good.

Morality, founded purely on sentiment, has inspired the attacks on vivisectors which in all confidence spread evil amongst men.

It is a surprising result of the great complexity of human affairs, that society is sometimes better served by wicked acts than by acts inspired by the most generous feelings. Thus extremely rigorous measures of repression are often more successful than the half-measures employed by humane and charitable administrators.

The intuitive theory of morality has had no greater success than utilitarianism. Even if the sentiment of society were a true basis of moral conduct, it fails in actual practice. On the other hand, although utility is the object of all morality, it is in most cases so difficult to determine what is really useful, that utilitarianism breaks down as the foundation of morality.

We must look elsewhere for principles which can guide us towards right conduct.

II

MORALITY AND HUMAN NATURE

Attempts to found morality on the laws of human nature—Kant's theory of moral obligation—Some criticisms of the Kantian theory—Moral conduct must be guided by reason

EVEN in antiquity, there were efforts to find a basis for morality other than the precepts of religion based on revelation, but the failure of such attempts has long been admitted. In the first chapter of *The Nature of Man*, I described such efforts to find a basis for morality in human nature itself. The Epicureans and the Stoics, although their doctrines were opposed, each claimed to set out from human nature. The principle is too vague for practical use, as human nature can be interpreted in very different fashions.

When several attempts to find a rational basis for morality had failed, Kant's theory appeared and was hailed by many as a real advance. None the less, it has not met with general approval and may be taken as a supreme instance of the failure to solve the great problem of morality by reason. I do not wish to deal with it at length, but a review of its main outlines is pertinent to my argument.

According to Kant, morality cannot be founded on the feeling of sympathy, nor can it have as its object the happiness of men. Nature would have been an unskilful workman were her object the happiness of human beings, for many lower animals have much more happiness. An inner law is the force compelling us to morality, and without that we should have to seek our guide in happiness.

Kant's doctrine is an intuitive theory of morality. It is based neither on sympathy nor on any inherent charity, which would make us covet happiness for our fellows, but solely on the consciousness of duty. Kant thought that the action of a man who wished to do good to his fellows was devoid of merit. Conduct was moral only in so far as it was obedience to the inner sense of duty. Schiller's epigram has thrown into relief this part of the great philosopher's theory, "When I take pleasure in doing good to my neighbour, I am uneasy, as I fear that I have been lacking in virtue."

In his criticism of Kant's system, Herbert Spencer drew a picture of a world inhabited by men who had no sympathy for their fellows and who did good to them against their natural instincts and only from a pure sense of duty. Spencer thought that such a world would be uninhabitable. Clearly, moral conduct, on the Kantian basis, could be followed only by exceptional persons, for most men follow their inclinations rather than any sense of duty. People of lower culture would accept kindnesses from others without caring whether the motive were kindness or a sense of duty, but highly civilised people would not endure service from those whom they knew to be acting against their instincts in obedience to a sense of duty. And so men would be driven to hide the real motives of their conduct, lest they should offend the sensibility of those towards whom their moral conduct was directed. Such cases, where the real motive is concealed, show how impossible it is to judge of conduct from the motives which may be supposed to have inspired it. As it is generally impossible to know whether some altruistic conduct has been inspired by kindness or has been performed as a duty, it is better to give up any attempt to appraise the springs of moral conduct.

Kant himself realised the need of some other standard for appraising human conduct. With such a purpose he arrived at his well-known maxim:—"Let your conduct be such that your motive might serve as a standard of universal application." To explain the maxim he gave a number of examples. A man who is without money and cannot pay a debt is in doubt as to whether he should promise to repay his creditor. According to Kant, he ought to ask himself what would be the result if such a promise were to be made under similar circumstances by everyone. It is plain that if such false promises became universal, they would cease to be believed and so would be impracticable in actual life. Kant's formula, therefore, would supply a rational basis for the discrimination of immoral conduct. In the case of theft it would operate as follows: if it became the custom for everyone to take whatever he wanted, private property and theft would simultaneously cease to exist. So also suicide is immoral, since if it became general the human race would cease to exist.

Kant, however, was looking at only one side of the problem. Moral conduct is frequently limited to an individual, and cannot be generalised for all humanity. Thus, for instance, if one about to sacrifice his life for the good of his fellows were to estimate his action according to Kant's formula, he would reach a conclusion similar to that in the case of suicide; if everyone were to sacrifice his life for others, no one would remain alive, and so, according to Kant, the sacrifice of one's life for the good of others would be an immoral act.

It is plain that in his search for a rational basis of morality, Kant found only a hollow form, void of any substantial body of morality. It is not enough that a moral man should take his consciousness of duty as a guide. He must know what would be the result of his acts. If it is immoral to make a false promise, it is because people would lose confidence in such promises, and confidence is necessary to our well-being. When the formula of Kant condemns theft, it is because, if theft became general, there could be no private property, and property is regarded as necessary to the well-being of men. Suicide is immoral, according to Kant, because it would lead to the disappearance of the human race, and human life is of course a good.

Kant tried to found his theory of morality on a rational basis which excluded the idea of the general good, but it was impossible for him to avoid it. His "practical reason," when it raised the consciousness of duty to a principle, should have pointed the goal towards which moral acts were to be directed. In this matter, I find that Kant's ideas are very vague, although extremely interesting.

The innate feeling of duty implies the *will* to pursue moral conduct. This will is independent of the circumambient conditions. Kant in his nebulous language explains this consideration as follows:—"Our reason informs us of a law to which all our maxims are subject, as if our will had created its own natural order of things. This law, then, is in the sphere of a nature which we do not know empirically but which the freedom of the will makes possible, a nature which is supra-sensible, but which from the practical point of view we make objective, because it is created by our will in virtue of our existence as rational beings. The difference between the laws of a nature to which the will is subject and a nature subject to the will subsists in this, that in the first the objects must be the causes which determine the will, whilst in the second, the will itself causes the objects so that the causality of the will resides exclusively in pure reason, pure reason being thus practical reason " (*Critique of Practical Reason*).

So far as I can follow the argument of Kant, it seems to me to imply that rational morality cannot be bound by human nature as it exists. I may perhaps interpret Kant's thought as if he had the intuition that the moral will was capable of modifying nature by subjecting it to its own laws.

On the other hand, several critics of Kant have attempted to improve his theory of morality by reconciling it with human nature as it actually exists. Vacherot,[1] for instance, has taken such an attitude in the most definite fashion. He insists that Kant "did not appreciate the capital importance of the object of the moral law. The problem which under the designation *summum bonum* absorbed the schools of antiquity plays a minor part in the Kantian theory. Kant should have recognised that human destiny is not limited to duty but must include happiness" (p. 316).

But what is this "happiness" which is to be the standard of human actions? To answer this Vacherot places himself in the position of those ancient philosophers whom I discussed in *The Nature of Man*. He makes his point absolutely clear. "What is the 'good' for any being? The attaining of its purpose. What is the purpose of a being? The simple development of its nature. Apply this to man and morality. When human nature is known by observation and analysis, the deduction can be made as to what is the purpose, and the good, and therefore the law of man. For the conception of the good necessarily in-

[1] *Essais de Philosophie critique*, Paris, 1864.

volves the idea of duty and of law to be imposed on the will. We have to fall back, then, on knowledge of man, but it must be complete knowledge, a recognition of the faculties, feelings, and inclinations that are peculiar to him and that distinguish him from animals" (p. 319). Here is a summary of this doctrine:—"Develop all our natural powers, subordinating those which are subsidiary to those which form the peculiar quality of human beings; this is the true economy of the little world we call human life; this is its purpose and this its law. The formula states in the most scientific and least doubtful form a very old truth, the foundation of all morality and the test of all its applications. If we seek to know what are justice, duty and virtue, we must look in the world itself, and not above or below it" (Op. 301).

Professor Paulsen, a more recent critic of Kant, comes to a similar conclusion.[1] He thinks that Kant should have modified his formula in some such way as follows:—" The laws of morality are rules which might serve for a natural legislation for human life; in other words, rules that, when they guided conduct according to natural law, would result in the preservation and supreme development of human life."

From whatever side we examine the problem of morality, we come to submit conduct to the laws of human nature. Sutherland, a modern author who discusses morality by the scientific method, defines morality as " conduct guided by rational sympathy." Such sympathy would not subordinate the chief good of others to an advantage less important but more immediate. Thus a mother may sympathise with her child when it has to take some unpleasant

[1] *System der Ethik*, 7th and 8th editions, vol. i, p. 199. Berlin 1906.

medicine; but if her sympathy be rational she will not let it interfere with the health of the child.

In the foregoing case, sympathy has to be controlled by medical knowledge. In moral conduct generally, reason must be the determining factor, whatever be the inspiring motive of the conduct, whether it come from sympathy or from the sense of duty. And thus morality in the last resort must be based on scientific knowledge.

III

INDIVIDUALISM

Individual morality—History of two brothers brought up in same circumstances, but whose conduct was quite different—Late development of the sense of life—Evolution of sympathy—The sphere of egoism in moral conduct—Christian morality—Morality of Herbert Spencer—Danger of exalted altruism

ALTHOUGH moral conduct refers specially to the relations between men, there exists a morality of the individual. As this latter is simpler, I shall consider it first in my investigation of rational morality.

When a man, seeking his individual happiness, gives way to his inclinations without restraint, he often comes to behave in a way that is generally regarded as immoral. Following his inclination, he may become idle and drunken. Idleness may depend on some irregularity of the brain, and may thus be as natural as is the wish to take drink in the case of a man to whom alcohol brings a feeling of well-being and gaiety. Why is it that idleness and alcoholism are immoral? Is it because they prevent the living of life in its completest and widest sense, according to the theory of Herbert Spencer? But it is precisely in this way that the adherents of the theory justify all kinds of excess without which fullness and width of life seem to them impossible.

Whilst vices such as idleness and drunkenness arise directly from qualities of the human constitution, they must be regarded as immoral because they prevent the completion of the ideal cycle of human life. I knew two brothers, almost the same age, subject to the same influences, and brought up in the same environment. None the less, their tastes and conduct were very different. The older brother, although very intelligent, during his college career devoted himself eagerly to bodily exercises and indulged in every way his inclination for pleasure. "As the chief end of life is happiness," he said, "one must try to get as much of it as possible," and so he got into the habit of visiting places where there was most amusement. Cards, good living, and women furnished for him the means of pleasure. As his ability was unusual, he passed his examinations almost without having worked. The example of his younger brother, always a devoted student, did not attract him. "It is all very well for you," he said, "as you find your happiness in work; as for me, I detest books, and I am happy only when I am giving myself up to pleasure. Everyone must take his own road to the goal of life." As a result, the health of the older brother was seriously affected by his mode of life. He acquired some disease of the circulatory system, had to face the end, and died at the age of fifty-six. The last years of his life were very unhappy, as the instinct of life developed in him extremely strongly. He was a victim of his own ignorance because when he was young he did not know that the sense of life would develop later on, and would become much stronger than in his youth. His brother was equally unaware of this fact, but, absorbed in scientific study, he kept himself apart from the indulgences of youth and lived a sober life. In this way he found that his strength and activity were fully preserved at a time of life when his older brother was already a physical wreck.

I have quoted this example, not to repeat the banal idea that a sober life is followed by a healthier old age than an intemperate life, but because I wish to insist on the importance of the development of the instinct of life in the course of each individual life. I see that this idea is very little known. I was present at the last moments of my older brother (he was called Ivan Ilyitch, and he was the subject of the famous story of Tolstoi: *The Death of Ivan Ilyitch*). Knowing that he was going to die from pyemia, at the age of forty-five, my brother preserved his great intelligence in all its clearness. As I sat by his bedside he told me his reflections in the most objective fashion possible. The idea of his death was for long very terrible to him, but " as we all die " he came to " resign himself, saying that after all there was only a quantitative difference between death at the age of forty-five and later on." This reflection, which relieved the moral sufferings of my brother, is none the less untrue. The sense of life is very different at different ages, and a man who lives beyond the age of forty-five experiences many sensations which he did not know before. There is a great evolution of the mind during the advance of age.

Even if we do not accept the existence of an instinct of natural death as the crown of normal life, we cannot deny that youth is only a preparatory stage and that the mind does not acquire its final development until later on. This conception should be the fundamental principle of the science of life and the guide for education and practical philosophy.

Individual morality consists of conduct permitting the accomplishment of the normal cycle of life and ending in a feeling of satisfaction as complete as possible and which can be reached only in advanced age. And so, when we see a man wasting his health and strength and youth, and thus making himself incapable of feeling the most complete pleasure in life, we call him immoral.

A man entirely isolated does not exist in nature. We are born weak and incapable of satisfying our needs and at once come into relations with the human being who feeds us and protects us. The child, although egoistic, becomes attached to his protector, and in this way the feeling of sympathy is born. Guided by this feeling as well as by the sense of his own interest, the child soon begins to employ his will in restraining some of his instincts, which, none the less, are quite natural. Thus, the fear of being deprived of food makes him obedient to his protectors. The child cannot complete his normal cycle without pursuing a certain moral conduct.

When he becomes adult, man experiences the instinctive need of relations with someone of the other sex. This need lays certain duties on him, and although the love of a young man is less egoistical than that of the child, it is far from presenting the characters of self-abnegation and sacrifice.

A young woman, after having passed through the usual cycle of life with her mother and with a man, becomes herself a mother. Maternal instinct furnishes her with certain rules of conduct, but this natural instinct is not enough to fulfil its object, that is to say, to rear the child until an age when it can live independently. Directed by a feeling of sympathy for her child, the young mother learns from women with more experience to ward off dangers from her child. In the first years, moral conduct on the part of the mother consists almost entirely in bringing up the child in a healthy way. For this purpose she must acquire much knowledge. If she remains ignorant, her conduct must be regarded as immoral.

So far as concerns the bringing up of a child, the moral problem is quite simple, because we are all agreed that the object is to rear the child to maturity in the healthiest possible condition. When the child exhibits any habits harmful to this object, although due to natural instincts, the mother applies her knowledge to restrain them without paying attention to the theory that happiness consists in the fulfilment of everything that is natural. When a child has passed through the perilous first period of its life, the mother has to ask what general object she is to follow in its education. She wishes her child to be as happy as possible. Here the conception of orthobiosis will serve her, and it will teach her that the greatest happiness consists in the normal evolution of the sense of life, leading to serene old age, and finally reaching the fulness of satiety of life. Man, who has passed his apprenticeship to life from his birth, with his protectors, and, later on, with persons of the other sex, inevitably acquires certain elements necessary for social life. Persuaded that in order to succeed in his individual life he must have help from his fellows, he learns to subdue his anti-social tendencies, at first in his own interests. Let me take an example of this. When a man has reached a certain stage of civilisation, it generally becomes impossible to him to supply his bodily wants without the help of persons less cultured than himself. He takes into his house one or more servants, with whom he enters into definite relations. He wishes for himself and those about him a normal life, such as I have described in *The Nature of Man*. To attain this it is indispensable in his own interest and in that of his family, that his domestic servants should be well treated. The health of the family very often depends on the conduct of the servants, who will follow conscientiously the hygienic rules only if they themselves are living in good conditions. The custom according to which the masters live in luxuriously furnished rooms, while their servants have mean quarters in the attics, is immoral from the point of view of the well-being of the masters themselves. The crowded servants' quarters are a nest of all sorts of infection, which may spread in the families of the masters. Very often people who think that they are following the rules of exact hygiene contract diseases without knowing that the infection has come from their servants.

Anger gives us another example. It is certainly harmful to the health, and so should be controlled in the interest of the bad-tempered person himself. Fits of rage are frequently followed by ruptures of blood-vessels, and by diabetes, and even cataracts have developed after some violent passion.

Luxurious habits are also well known to be harmful to the health. Heavy meals, evenings passed in the theatre and in society may seriously affect activity of the organs. Moreover, the luxury of some people is often the cause of misery to others. The knowledge that luxurious habits shorten life and prevent man from reaching the greatest happiness may warn people against luxury better than the appeal to the feeling of sympathy.

As it is a fact that most men guide their lives generally from egoistic motives, any theory of morality which is to be put into practice must reckon seriously with this factor. All other systems have recognised it. In the Sermon on the Mount, which is a summary of Christian morality, each moral act is recognised on the ground that it will bring some reward or obviate some punishment. "Rejoice," said Jesus, "and be exceeding glad; for great is your reward in heaven" (Matt. v., 12). "Take heed that ye do not your alms before men, to be seen of them; otherwise ye have no reward of your Father which is in heaven" (Matt. vi., 1). "That thine alms may be in secret; and thy Father which seeth in secret himself shall reward thee openly" (Matt. vi., 4). "Judge not, that ye be not judged" (Matt. vii., 1). "But if ye forgive not men their trespasses, neither will your Father forgive your trespasses" (Matt. vi., 15). Jesus had no high opinion of the influence of altruism on human conduct.

Herbert Spencer in his treatise on morality (*The Data of Ethics*) also insists that laws of conduct, to be of general application, must not require men to make too great sacrifices, as otherwise the best teaching would remain a dead letter. He imagines, however, that in the future the human race will be so much improved that moral conduct will become instinctive, needing no compulsion. The English philosopher presents a view of the future of the human race totally at variance with the Kantian conception. Instead of human beings becoming filled with a sense of duty opposed to their natural instincts, the world will be peopled with men acting morally from inclination, so making the world delightful.

The ideal is so far removed from existing conditions that the possibility of its attainment is hardly worth considering. It is probable that a world whose inhabitants had the feeling of sympathy very highly developed would not be so delightful. For sympathy is generally a reaction against evil. When evil disappears, sympathy would be not merely useless, but annoying and harmful.

George Eliot in *Middlemarch* describes a young woman

INDIVIDUALISM

enthusiastically anxious to do good to her fellows. When she came to live in a village, she made great plans to succour its poor. Her disillusion and annoyance were great when she found that the villagers were quite comfortably off, and had no need of her charity.

John Stuart Mill in his *Autobiography* relates that when he was young he dreamed of reforming society and making everyone happy. But when he asked himself if the accomplishment of his beautiful ideas would make him happy, he was compelled to answer "No!" and this discovery plunged the young philosopher into a lamentable condition. He described himself as quite overcome, all that supported him in life crumbling away. His happiness could lie only in the constant pursuit of his object, and the charm seemed broken, because if attainment were not to please him, how could the means be of any interest to him? It seemed to him that nothing was left to which he could dedicate his life.

As it is highly probable that with the advance of civilisation the greatest evils of humanity will become lessened, and may even disappear, the sacrifices to be made will also become less. Now that there is a serum which protects against plague, there is no room for the heroism of the doctors who used to incur the greatest danger in fighting epidemics. Until lately doctors used to risk their life in treating the throats of diphtheric patients. A young doctor who was a friend of mine, of high ability and promise, died from diphtheria contracted under these conditions. He met his death, in isolation from his friends in case of infecting them, with the utmost heroism. Now that the antidiphtheric serum has been discovered, such heroism would be unnecessary. The advance of science has removed the occasion of such sacrifices.

It is now very long since there has been opportunity for the heroism which steeled the hand of Abraham to sacrifice his only son to his religion. Human sacrifice, based on the highest morality, has become more and more rare, and will finally disappear. Rational morality, although it may admire such conduct, has no use for it. So also, it may foresee a time when men will be so highly developed that instead of being delighted to take advantage of the sympathy of their fellows, they will refuse it absolutely. Neither the Kantian idea of virtue, doing good as a pure duty, nor that of Herbert Spencer, according to which men have an instinctive need to help their fellows, will be realised in the future. The ideal will rather be that of men who will be self-sufficient and who will no longer permit others to do them good.

IV

ORTHOBIOSIS

Human nature must be modified according to an ideal—Comparison with the modification of the constitution of plants and of animals—Schlanstedt rye—Burbank's plants—The ideal of orthobiosis—The immorality of ignorance—The place of hygiene in the social life—The place of altruism in moral conduct—The freedom of the theory of orthobiosis from metaphysics

As I have shown in *The Nature of Man*, the human constitution as it exists to-day, being the result of a long evolution and containing a large animal element, cannot furnish the basis of rational morality. The conception which has come down from antiquity to modern times, of a harmonious activity of all the organs, is no longer appropriate to mankind. Organs which are in course of atrophy must not be reawakened, and many natural characters which perhaps were useful in the case of animals must be made to disappear in men.

Human nature, which, like the constitutions of other organisms, is subject to evolution, must be modified according to a definite ideal. Just as a gardener or stock raiser is not content with the existing nature of the plants and animals with which he is occupied, but modifies them to suit his purposes, so also the scientific philosopher must not think of existing human nature as immutable, but must try to modify it for the advantage of mankind.

As bread is the chief article in human food, attempts to improve cereals have been made for a very long time. Rimpau made one of the greatest steps in this direction when he introduced into cultivation a variety of rye known as Schlanstedt rye, now fairly abundant in France and Germany. Rimpau set himself the task of producing a variety with the longest ears and containing many and heavy grains. Having conceived his ideal, he began to seek out what was nearest to it in a very large number of examples of rye. After patient and continued labour, using careful selection and cross-fertilisation, Rimpau succeeded in making the new variety, and so did a great service to mankind.

Burbank,[1] an American horticulturist, has recently gained a wide reputation because of his improvements of useful plants. He has produced a new kind of potato which has raised the value of potato crops in the United States by about £3,500,000 per annum. Burbank cultivated great numbers of fruit trees, flowers, and all kinds of plants, with the object of increasing their utility. One of his objects was to produce varieties which could resist dry conditions, which reproduced rapidly and so forth. He has modified the nature of plants to such an extent that he has cactus plants and brambles without thorns. The succulent leaves of the former provide an excellent food for cattle, whilst the absence of thorns in the latter makes their pleasant fruit more suitable for gardens. Burbank has enormously improved the production of stoneless plums, and has very much reduced the price of many bulbs and lilies by increasing their productivity.

To obtain such results much knowledge and a long period of time were necessary. To modify the nature of

[1] De Vries, in *Biologisches Centralblatt*, 1906, Sept. 1st, p. 609.

plants it was necessary to understand them well. To frame the new ideal of the plant it was necessary not only to have an exact conception of what was wanted, but to find out if the qualities of the plants in question furnished any hope of realising it.

The methods which have been successful in the case of plants and animals must be much modified for application to the human race. In the case of human beings the selection and cross-breeding which were imposed upon rye and plum trees are not possible, but, at the same time, the ideal of human nature, towards which mankind ought to press, may be formed. In our opinion this ideal is orthobiosis, that is to say, the development of the human life so that it passes through a long period of old age in active and vigorous health, leading to the final period in which there shall be present a sense of satiety of life, and a wish for death. I do not think that the ideal should be that of Herbert Spencer, a simple prolongation of human life. When the instinct of death comes at a not very late period of life, there would be no inconvenience in shortening the life, if death did not come soon after the appearance of the instinct. Probably this would be the only case where suicide was justified in the conception of orthobiosis.

The foregoing is the case of an action in conformity with the ideal, but quite contrary to human nature as it is at present. A similar contradiction appears in reproduction. Man came from animals amongst which unlimited reproduction was an important factor in the preservation of the species, as it allowed the species to survive under all sorts of bad conditions, such as diseases, combats, attacks of enemies, and changes of climate. Although man, according to the laws of human nature, is capable of reproducing extremely rapidly, the ideal of his happiness makes a restriction of this power necessary. Thus orthobiosis, based upon knowledge of human nature, would set limits to a function which is perhaps the most natural of all. The restriction which is already partially adopted will come more and more into operation as the struggle against diseases, the prolongation of human life, and the suppression of war make progress. It will be one of the chief means of diminishing the most brutal forms of the struggle for existence, and of increasing moral conduct amongst mankind.

Just as Rimpau began to study the nature of plants before trying to realise his ideal, so also varied and profound knowledge is the first requisite for the ideal of moral conduct. It is necessary not only to know the structure and function of the human organism, but to have exact ideas on human life as it is in society. Scientific knowledge is so indispensable for moral conduct that ignorance must be placed among the most immoral acts. A mother who rears her child in defiance of good hygiene, from want of knowledge, is acting immorally towards her offspring, notwithstanding her feeling of sympathy. And this also is true of a Government which remains in ignorance of the laws which regulate human life and human society.

It must be well understood that I am not here thinking of written knowledge, set down in treatises and volumes. Rimpau and Burbank went outside manuals of botany to obtain their knowledge. Besides books, wide ideas on the practice of life are required to direct aright the conduct of men. A doctor who has just finished his studies at the hospital, notwithstanding all his knowledge, is not yet sufficiently trained to be a good practitioner. He must acquire the habit of treating patients, and for this years are required. So also is it with regard to the practical applications of the principles of morality. The regulation of conduct requires profound knowledge both theoretical and practical, and men selected to frame or to apply laws of morality must have this double qualification. If the human race come to adopt the principles of orthobiosis, a considerable change in the qualities of men of different ages will follow. Old age will be postponed so much that men of from sixty to seventy years of age will retain their vigour, and will not require to ask assistance in the fashion now necessary. On the other hand, young men of twenty-one years of age will no longer be thought mature or ready to fulfil functions so difficult as taking a share in public affairs. The view which I set forth in *The Nature of Man* regarding the danger which comes from the present interference of young men in political affairs has since then been confirmed in the most striking fashion.

It is easily intelligible that in the new conditions such modern idols as universal suffrage, public opinion, and the *referendum*, in which the ignorant masses are called on to decide questions which demand varied and profound knowledge, will last no longer than the old idols. The progress of human knowledge will bring about the replacement of such institutions by others, in which applied morality will be controlled by the really competent persons. I permit myself to suppose that in these times, scientific training will be much more general than it is just now, and that it will occupy the place which it deserves in education and in life.

It is equally clear that if a mother is to act morally with regard to her child, she must teach herself properly. In place of mythology and literature, she must learn hygiene and all that relates to the rational rearing of children. So, also, in the education of men, the study of the exact sciences must occupy by far the most important place. Then only will moral conduct and scientific knowledge begin to unite. An ignorant mother will bring up a child very badly notwithstanding all her good will and her affection. A doctor, however imbued with strong sympathy for his patients, could do them much harm if he had not the appropriate knowledge. Are not politicians open to the reproach from the point of view of morality that very often through ignorance they do the very worst evil in public administration? With the progress of knowledge, moral conduct and useful conduct will become more and more closely identified.

I have been reproached because in my system the health of the body occupies too large a place. It cannot be otherwise, because health certainly plays the chief part in existence. Notwithstanding his pessimism, Schopenhauer was convinced that health was the greatest treasure, a treasure before which everything else yielded. In many religions care of the health is laid down amongst the chief duties. Although many scientific men do not hold the opinion that circumcision was ordained for hygienic reasons, it is certain that hygiene was extremely important in the Jewish religion. It is only in Christianity, which despises the human body, that hygiene is excluded from the religious code, as in the words of Jesus:—

"Take no thought for your life, what ye shall eat, or what ye shall drink; nor yet for your body, what ye shall put on. Is not the life more than meat, and the body than raiment?" (Matt. vi., 25). As for long ages hygiene was very imperfectly known, it is not surprising that it played a small part in human affairs. Probably the objection to the importance that I assign to it in orthobiosis is a relic from the old order of things. Now, however, the situation is different. Bacteriology has placed hygiene on a scientific foundation, so that the latter is now one of the exact sciences. It has now become necessary to give it the chief place in applied morality as it is the branch of knowledge that teaches how men ought to live.

It has been objected that I have left no place for altruism in my system.[1] Certainly I have tried to find an egoistic basis for moral conduct, as I have shown above. I think, however, that the wish to live according to the ideal of orthobiosis and to make others live a normal life would be a powerful agency in improving social life, in preventing mutual damage, and promoting mutual help. Such a motive, within the reach of persons whose altruistic feelings are not specially strong, must largely extend moral conduct amongst human beings, and even although in future such manifestations of high morality as the sacrifice of life and health will become wholly or nearly wholly useless, I think that for the present there is still room for altruism. The practical application of scientific knowledge already gained admits much self-denial and good feeling. Struggle against prejudices of all kinds and the development and diffusion of sound ideas require a conduct very highly altruistic.

The fears of my opponents are still less justified when we reflect that the feelings of sympathy and of cohesion must play a large part in the business of helping the evolution of man towards the goal of normal life.

Although our actual knowledge already provides a basis of rational morality, it may be admitted that in the future, if science continues its forward march, the rules of moral conduct will become still more improved. There will

[1] Dr. Grasset, "La fin de la vie" in the *Revue de philosophie*, Aug. 1st, 1903.

be no ground for reproaching me for a blind faith in the all-powerfulness of science. Much more trust can be given to one who has faithfully carried out his promises, than to one who has promised much and fulfilled nothing. Science has already justified the hopes which have been placed in it. It has saved people from the most terrible diseases, and has made life much easier. On the other hand, religions, which demand an uncritical faith as the means of curing the ills which afflict humanity, have not fulfilled their promises.

The reproach that I preach blind faith in the progress of science, destined to replace religious faith, is unjust, because my faith depends on a confidence that science has already deserved. Equally unjust is the reproach that I have built my system on a partly metaphysical principle. According to M. Parodi,[1] the hypothesis of physiological old age and of natural death seem to "involve the idea of a natural duration of human life, which, however, from accidental reasons man does not complete at present. M. Metchnikoff repeatedly uses the expression 'normal cycle.' Now do we not see here the surreptitious repetition of the old teleological conception of nature, although at first he so energetically disavowed it? It is the belief that the species is a necessary reality, corresponding to a definite type of its own, in fact a special design of nature; that nature, to guide herself, had an ideal which circumstances could mistake or degrade, but which had to be restored to its perfect form? Otherwise, why does he insist that there must be a condition of perfect and stable equilibrium between individual and environment? that there is a normal cycle and that it must be possible to harmonise the disharmonies?"

I can show easily that all these objections rest upon a

[1] "Morale et biologie," *Revue philosophique*, 1904, vol. lviii, p. 125.

simple misunderstanding. I have never conceived of the existence of any ideal of nature or of the inevitable necessity of transforming disharmonies to harmonies. I have no knowledge of the " designs " and " motives " of nature; I have never taken my stand on metaphysical ground. I have not the remotest idea if nature has any ideal and if the appearance of man on the earth were a part of such an ideal. What I have spoken of is the ideal of man corresponding to the need to ward off the great evils of old age as it is now, and of death as we see it around us. I have said, moreover, that human nature, that collection of complex features of multiple origin, contains certain elements which may be used to modify it according to our human ideal. I have done nothing but what the horticulturist does when he finds in the nature of plants elements which suggest to him to try and make new and improved races. Just as the constitution of some plum trees contains elements which make it possible to produce plums without stones which are pleasanter to eat, so also in our own nature there exist characters which make it possible to transform our disharmonious nature into a harmonious one, in accordance with our ideal, and able to bring us happiness. I have not the smallest idea what ideal nature may have on the subject of plums, but I know very well that man has such designs and such an ideal as form a point of departure for the transformation of the nature of plums. Substitute man for the plum tree and you are at my point of view. When I have spoken of the normal cycle of life or of physiological old age, I have used the words normal and physiological only in relation to our ideal of the human constitution. I might just as well have said that a cactus without thorns is the normal cactus in the conditions where it was desired to obtain a succulent plant useful as food for cattle. The words "normal" and "physiological" seemed to me more convenient than such a phrase as "in correspondence with human ideals."

I am so little convinced of the existence of any disposition of nature to transform our ills into goods, and our disharmonies into harmonies, that it would not surprise me if such an ideal were never reached. Even in unmetaphysical circles it is said that nature has the intention of preserving the species at the expense of the individual. The ground of this is that the species survives the individual. On the other hand, very many species have completely disappeared. Amongst these species were animals very highly organised, such as some anthropoid apes (*Dryopithecus*, etc.). As nature has not spared these, how can we be certain that she is not ready to deal with the human race in the same way. It is impossible for us to know the unknown, its plans and motives. We must leave nature on one side and concern ourselves with what is more congruous with our intelligence.

Our intelligence informs us that man is capable of much, and for this reason we hope that he may be able to modify his own nature and transform his disharmonies into harmonies. It is only human will that can attain this ideal.

INDEX

ABELARD, 273
Abraham, use of soured milk, 171
Ackermann, Mde., 237
Actinosphærium, degeneration in, 14
Adanson, on age of Baobab-tree, 98
Adrenaline, effect of, 121
Agave, duration of life of, 100
Aged, treatment of in uncivilised countries, 1, 2
Alcohol and longevity, 91, 92
Algeria, ostriches at, 76, 78, 79
Altruism, 331
Ambard, Dr., on Mde. Robineau, 7
Anæmia, of brain, and sleep, 122
  use of serums in, 149
André, M., use of serums in anæmia, 149
Anger, 321
Annandale, Nelson, on age of anemones, 48
Annuals, change to biennials or perennials, 100
  death of, 102
Antelopes, excreta of, 66
Anthropoids, mental characters of, 191 et seq.
Antiseptics, use of, in intestinal putrefaction, 156
Ants, 220, 221
Apes, anthropoid, mental characters of, 191 et seq.
  relationship to man, 184, 185
Arabs, use of milk by, 174
Aristotle, 132
Arteries, sclerosis of, in the aged, 31
Ascidians, social, 219
Ashworth, Mr., on age of anemones, 48
Atheroma, in the aged, 30
Atrophy, of cells, 26
  of muscles, 28

Auditory apparatus, rudimentary organism, 188
Augsburg, elixir of life, 138
Auto-intoxication, from intestinal putrefaction, 69
  in plants, 107
  sleep, due to, 120

Babinsky, Dr., hysteria a relic from apes, 209
Balkan States, centenarians frequent in, 90
Baobab-tree, age of, 98
Barth, Dr., definition of somnambulism, 206
Batrachia, longevity of, 50
Bats, intestinal flora of, 80, 81
Bees, 49, 220, 226
Beetroot, perennial variety of, 100
Belgium, old age pensions, 4
Bélonovsky, M., on serums in anæmia, 148
Bélonowsky, Dr., on Bulgarian bacillus, 170
Berthelot, on dragon-tree of Orotava, 96
Bertrand, M. G., on sorbose fermentation, 106
Bertrand and Weisweiler, on *Bacillus bulgaris*, 179
Besredka, M., on blood serums, 148, 149
Bielschowsky, biographer of Goethe, 269
Blanchard, E., on age of carp, 50
Birds, intestinal flora of, 76, 79
  longevity of, 52
Blindness, 248, 257
Bloch, Dr. I., on Schopenhauer, 247

INDEX

Blood-vessels, hardening of, in the old, 31
Bodio, on infant mortality, 85
Boerhave, on gerokomy, 136
Bones, degeneration of, 29, 30
Bordet, M. J. M., on serums, 148
Botulism, poison of, 70, 82
Bouchard, M., on disinfection of intestines, 156
Bouchet, M., on constipation after parturition, 68
Bourneville, M., on effects of extirpation of thyroid, 34
Boveri, M., produced atherana by nicotine, 32
Bone, marrow, in old age, 37
Botryllus, 219
Boutroux, definition of morality, 303
Bradyfagy, 159
Brain, anæmia of, as cause of sleep, 122
Brehm, on age of cattle, 55
Brettes, criticism of " rudimentary organs," 186
Bricon, M., on effects of extirpation of thyroid, 34
Brigand, Calabrian, fear of death, 194, 195
Brillat-Savarin, quotation from, 126
Brown-Séquard, specific for long life, 139, 277
Brudzinsky, M., on use of lactic microbes, 181
Buddha, on pessimism, 233, 247
Buehler, Dr., on cause of old age, 16
Buffon, on duration of life, 40, 50
Bulgarian bacillus, 178, 179, 180, 181, 182
Bunge, on relation between growth and longevity, 42
Burbank, American horticulturist, 326, 328
Butterflies, longevity of, 57
Bütschli, O., on life of cells, 15
Byron, 239, 247, 295

Cachexia, after extirpation of thyroid gland, 34
Caeca, of vertebrates, 60 *et seq.*
Cagliostro, elixir of life, 138
Calomel, as an intestinal antiseptic, 158
and syphilis, 146
Camphor, as an intestinal antiseptic, 156

Canary Islands, 96
Cancalon, Dr., on instinct of death, 128, 129
Cancer, and cleanliness, 144
Candolle, A. de, on cypresses of Mexico, 98
on age of trees, 99
Cantacuzène, M., on blood serums, 148
Capital punishment, 305
Carlyle, on " Werther," 265
Castration, effects of, 272
Cats, longevity of, 56
Cattle, longevity of, 55
Celibacy, and education of women, 224
Cell reproduction, rate of, 16
Centenarians, 4, 5, 86, 88, 89, 175, 176
Charcot, on sterilised food, 162, 163
on hysteria, 202
Charron, M., on putrefactive poisons, 69
Chemin, M., on centenarians, 88, 89
Chimpanzee, 185, 192, 193
China, Emperor Chi-Hoang-Ti and immortality, 137
Chopin, a degenerate, 134
Christian morality, 321, 330
Chromophags, action of, 25
Claparède, E., on theory of sleep, 123, 124, 125
Cleanliness, and increase of life, 144
Clergymen, increasing duration of life of, 142
Coffee and longevity, 92
Cohausen, on gerokomy, 137
Cohendy, Dr. M., on Bulgarian bacillus, 178
on intestinal flora, 78, 79
on intestinal putrefaction, 168
on thymol as a disinfectant, 157
Collectivism, 228
Colon, absorption in, 64
Constipation, evil results of, 67, 68, 69
Cooking, effect of, on microbes in food, 162
Copenhagen, suicide in, 3
Coral polyps, 216
Cornaro, 91
Cossacks, and biennial rye, 100
Cretinism, compared with senility, 32
Crœsus, 197
Cryptogams, life of, 99

INDEX

Cursorial birds, intestinal flora of, 76
Cypress, age of, 98
Czerny, M., on absorption in colon, 64
— on cancer, 144

D'Alton, and Goethe, 280
Dalyell, old anemone of, 48
Dana, on *monstrilla*, 115
Darwin, on fear, 195
David, King, 136
Death, instinct of, 128, 129
— natural, 94, 109, 119
— sensations at approach of, 126, 127, 130
Debreuil, Ch., on defecation in rheas, 76
— on excreta of antelopes, 66
Degenerates, famous, 134
Delage, Yves, criticism of instinct of death, 128
— on function of large intestines, 65, 66
Demange, M., on old age, 119
Denmark, suicide in, 3, 237
Descent of man, 184
Despotism, and socialism, 230
de Vries, H., on duration of life of plants, 104
— on prolongation of life of plants, 100
— on natural death in plants, 101
Diet and longevity, 46
Digestive system and senility, 59
Diplogaster, mother killed by larvæ, 111
Diphtheria, 323
Disease, and shortening of life, 145 *et seq.*
Doctors, lady, 225
Dodo, 213
Dogs, longevity of, 55
Dostoiewsky, quotation from, 2
Doyen, M., operation on double monsters, 216
Dragon-tree, of Orotava, 96, 97, 98
Drakenberg, age of, 87
Drunkenness, and morality, 317
Dryopithecus, 334
Ducks, old, 11
Duering, on pessimism, 248
Durand-Fardel, M., on atheroma, 30
Duration of life, in animals, 39 *et seq.*, 133

Eagles, intestinal flora of, 82
Ecclesiastes, quotation from, 233
Eckermann, narrative of Goethe's last years, 271, 274, 279
Egoism, 227, 306, 331
Egyptian milk, 105
Eimer, Th., on intestines of bats &c., 62, 63
Einhorn, Dr., on bradyfagy, 159
Elective Affinities, Goethe's, 273
Elephants, 9, 54, 83, 197
Eliot, George, 322
Elixir vitæ, 138
Ellenberger, on digestion in horse, 78
Enriquez, on infusoria, 13
Ephemeridæ, duration of life of, 113, 118
Epicureans, 309
Epiphyses of bones, as giving period of growth, 40
Ermenghem, van, on botulism, 70
Errera, Dr., on cause of sleep, 121
Eudoxia, 218
Ewald, on absorption in colon, 64
Exhaustion, as cause of plant death, 104, 107
Extinction of animals, 213
Eye, in old age, 36

Fatigue, Weichardt on cause of, 123
"*Faust*" and Goethe, 283 *et seq.*
Favorsky, Dr., on botulism, 82
Fear, analysis of, 194
Fecundity and duration of life, 43, 44, 45, 57, 58
Feinkind, case of somnambulism quoted from, 204
Femininist movement, 224
Fermentation, cause of, 105
Fertility and longevity, 44, 45
Fish, longevity of, 50
Flamans, M., 5
Fletcher, on chewing, 159
Flora, of intestines, poisonous effect of, 70, 73 *et seq.*, 151 *et seq.*
Flourens, on duration of life, 40, 84
Foà, on use of soured milk in Africa, 172
Food, evil effects of putrefaction in, 163
Fouard, M., on soured milk, 180
Fürbbinger, on Brown-Séquard's emulsions, 139

INDEX

Gautier, A., on leucomaines, 121
Gegenbaur, on intestinal tract, 60, 61
Genius and sexual power, 272
Gerokomy, 136
Gessner, on age of pike, 50
Gestation and longevity, 42
Giacomini, on Harderian gland, 189
Gibbons, 192, 198
Goebel, on duration of life of prothalli, 101, 102
Goethe, 260-300, 305
"Goose-skin," 196
Gorilla, strength of, 192
Griesbach, on sense of touch in blind, 257
Grigoroff, on Bulgarian yahourth, 175, 178
Grindon, on age of sheep, 55
Guinon, Dr., on a case of hysteria, 203
Gurney, J. H., on longevity of birds, 51, 79

HAECKEL, on medical selection, 134
Haffkine, M., 112
Hair, 17, 18
Halictus, a solitary bee, 226
Haller, on human longevity, 84, 132
Hamlet, quotation from, 239
Hannibal, his elephants swim the Rhone, 197
Harderian gland, 189
Hartmann, 235, 241
Harvey, on Parr, 87
Hayem, Prof., on use of lactic acid, 169, 173
Heart, diseases of, and syphilis, 145, 146
Hegesias, and suicide, 234
Heile, on absorption in colon, 64
Heim, on microbes in milk, 176
Heim, Prof., on Alpine accidents, 130
Heine, 236, 240
Hermippus, and gerokomy, 137
Herter, Dr., experiments on lactic acid in dogs, 167
Hertwig, R., on *Actinosphærium*, 14
Hildebrand, on duration of life of plants, 101, 102
Hippocrates, 132
Hofmeister, on digestion in horse, 74
Honey-ant, 222

Horse, cæcum, 62
 digestion, 74
 use of serum, 147
Horsley, Sir V., on effects of extirpation of thyroid, 34
Horst, on a somnambulistic soldier, 203
Hufeland, quotation from "Macrobiotique," 137
Hugo, V., and sexuality, 277
Humboldt, on dragon-tree of Orotava, 96
 on longevity of parrots, 52
Hunger, compared with sleep, 125
Huxley, on character of Orang, 193
Hygiene, and old age, 141, 142, 143
Hypnotism, of a crowd on individuals, 210
Hysteria, analysis of, 200 *et seq.*
 in monkeys, 208

IBSEN, and sexuality, 277
Idleness, 316
Immortality, Chinese beverage for, 137, 138
Incubation, duration of, compared with longevity, 41, 42
India, government of, and age of elephants, 54
Individualism, 316
Individuality, 212 *et seq.*
Infusoria, death of, 95
 senescence of, 13
Insects, ages of, 49
 social, 220 *et seq.*
Instinct, of death, 128, 129
 maternal, 319, 320, 329
 social, 306
Intestine, large, 59, 65, 67, 151
Intuitive theory of morality, 305

JACOBSON, organ of, 187
Javal, Dr., on characters of the blind, 257, 259
Jenner, effect of vaccination on mortality rate, 144
Josué, M., artificial production of atheroma, 32
Jousset, Dr., on difference between man and apes, 184

KANT, 309, 310
Kautsky, on socialism, 229, 230
Kentigern, age of, 87

INDEX

Kephir, 171, 172, 173
Khoury, M., on ferment of Egyptian milk, 105
Kocher, Dr., on effects of extirpation of thyroid gland, 33
Kocher, Prof., case of removal of large intestine, 152, 153
Kölliker, on degeneration of muscles, 27
Koppenfels, on character of gorilla, 194
Koumiss, 172
Kowalevsky, Sophie, 225
Kowalevsky, analysis of pessimism, 241, 255
Kukula, experiments on intestinal poisons, 69, 70
Kwass, 166

LACTIC BACILLI, and putrefaction in intestine, 168
Laignel-Lavastine, M., criticism of neuronophagy, 20
Lankester, Sir E. Ray, on longevity, 12, 56
Lao-Tsé, and immortality, 137
Laud, Archbishop, old tortoise of, 51
Lautschenberger, on absorption in colon, 64
Lavater, Goethe's letter to, 268
Laws aiding the aged, 3, 4
"Leben," Egyptian, 105, 171, 177, 178
Le Bon, G., on hysteria in crowds, 209
Lenau, M., 236
Lenthéric, on elephants swimming, 197
Leopardi, G., pessimistic poet, 235, 236, 247
Le Play, M., on putrefactive poisons, 69
Léri, M., on senile brain, 20
Lermontoff, 236
Leucomaines, as cause of sleep, 121
Levaillant, on longevity of parrots, 52
Lewes, G. H., on Goethe, 273, 290, 292, 298
Lexis, on duration of human life, 85
Life, duration of, in animals, 39 et seq.
Life, prolongation of human, 132, et seq.
"sense" of, 260

Lima, Dr., on use of soured milk in Africa, 172, 174
Lloyd, M., old anemone of, 47
London Zoological Gardens, 51, 81
Longevity, in animal kingdom, 47 et seq.
human, 84 et seq.
rules for, 141
in sexes, 44
theories of, 39
Lorand, Dr., on ductless glands, 32
Love, Goethe and, 272
Loewenberg, Dr., on Mde. Robineau, 7
Luxury, 321

MACFADYEN, Nencki and Mde. Sieber, on digestion, 153, 161
Macrophags, 25, 147
Mailaender, 235, 255
Malaquin, M., on *Monstrilla*, 116, 117
Male rotifers, death of, 114, 115
Malthus, theory of, 214
Mammals, longevity of, 53
Mammary glands, in males, 186
Man, compared with apes, 184, 185
natural death of, 119 et seq.
longevity of, 84 et seq.
Manouélian, M., on neuronophagy, 21, 22
Marinesco, M., on neuronophogs, 19
Marrow of the bones, in old age, 37
Marsiliaceae, duration of life of prothallus, 99
Martin, on Gibbons, 192
Massart, on cause of death in plants, 102, 109
Massol, Prof., 178
Mastication, and intestinal putrefaction, 160
Matchinsky, M., on atrophy of ovary, 26
Maternal instinct, 319, 320
Mauclaire, M., operations on large intestine, 153, 154, 155
Maumus, M., on digestion in caeca, 61
Mauritius, giant tortoise from, 12
Maupas, M., on infusoria, 13
Maya, 178
Mayers, on Chinese elixir, 138
Meconium, appearance of microbes in, 161

INDEX

Medical selection, 134
Mesnet and Mottet, Drs., cases of hysteria, 203
Mice, duration of life, 41, 43, 56
Michaelis, on muscles of monkeys, 185
Microbes, as cause of senility, 73
    in food, 162, 163
    passage through intestinal walls, 71
Middlemarch, G. Eliot's, 322
Milk, importance of boiling, 177, 178
    microbes of disease in, 177
    putrefaction and fermentation of, 167
    use of soured milk, 181, 182
Mill, J. S., 323
Milne-Edwards, H., on laws of duration of life, 42
Minot, Prof., on cause of old age, 16
Moa, 213
Moebius, on Goethe, 271
    on Schopenhauer, 255
Molluscs, ages of, 48
Mongols, hair in old, 17
Monkeys, longevity of, 83
Monsters, double, 216
Monstrilla, life-history of, 115, 116, 117
Montefiore, Sir M., 91
Morality, Christian, 321
    definitions of, 303
    Kantian, 309, 310, 311, 312
    science and, 301 *et seq.*
Mortality rates of old persons, 142, 143
Moses, use of soured milk, 171
Mosso, on fear, 194, 196
Muscles, degeneration of, 9, 26, 27
Myxomycetes, 215

NAEGELI, on age of trees, 99
Nails, growth of, in the old, 18
Naphthaline, as an intestinal antiseptic, 156
Nature, human, 325
Nausenne, Mde., cause of longevity, 141
Negroes, longevity of, 88
Neisser, Prof., on protection against syphilis, 146
Nematodes, death of, 111
Nemertines, life-history of *Pilidium* of, 109 *et seq.*
Nencki and Sieber, on digestion, 153, 161, 169

Neurononhags, 19, 20, 21, 22, 23, 24
Nicotine, use of in experimental production of atheroma, 32
Nietzsche, criticism of Socialism, 230
Nogueira, M., on use of soured milk in Africa, 172, 174

OBSTACLES, sense of, 258
Old age, Goethe and, 279 *et seq.*
Olympian, Goethe as an, 269
Optimism, foundation of, 256
    Goethe's transformation to, 269, 270 *et seq.*
Orang-outan, 185, 193
Orotava, dragon-tree of, 96
Orstein, Dr., on centenarians in Greece, 90
Orthobiosis, 212, 325 *et seq.*
Ossetes, use of soured milk, 173
Osteoclasts, 30
Ostrich, defecation of, 76
Oustalet, M., on longevity of vertebrates, 46
Ovary, atrophy of, 26
Owls, intestinal flora of, 83
Ownership, collective, 229, 230

PARODI, on old age, 332
Parr, Thomas, 87
Parrots, duration of life, 41
    scanty intestinal flora of, 79
Pasquier, Dr. du, on constipation, 67
Pasteur, discovery of lactic microbe, 105, 167
Paulsen, criticism of Kant, 314
Pensions, old age, 3, 4, 133
Pessimism, 129, 233, 234, 239, 241, 249, 266
Pessimist, study of life-history of a, 249 *et seq.*
Pflüger, on longevity, 93
Phagocytes, 18, 19
Phagocytosis, examples of, 25, 37
Phalansteries, 229
Pilidium, 109 *et seq.*
Pitres, M., hysteric patients of, 200
Plague, 323
Plants, death of, 99, 103
Plasmodia, of Myxomycetes, 215, 216
Pleurotrocha haffkini, 112, 113
Pochon, Dr., experiments on use of lactic bacilli, 169
Poehl, Dr., on spermine, 139, 140
Pohl, Dr., on growth of hair, 17, 18
Ponogenes, as cause of sleep, 120

INDEX

Potatoes, improved by Burbank, 326
Poushkin, 236
Predestination, and plants, 103
Preyer, Dr., on *Ponogenes*, 120
Prichard, on longevity of negroes, 88
Productivity compared with fecundity, 57, 58
Prostokwacha, 172, 176
Prolongation of life, 132 *et seq.*
Prothalli, life of, 99
Psychids, death of, 117
Ptolemy, fear of Hegesias' philosophy, 235
Punishment, capital, 305
Purgatives, use of, in intestinal putrefaction, 157
Putrefaction, intestinal, 151 *et seq.*, 161, 163, 164

QUÉTELET, on stature of the aged, 9

RABBIT, fecundity of, 58
Ravens, absence of putrefaction in intestines of, 75
Reagents, action of, in distorting tissues, 20
Renouvier, C., on his own death, 127
Reproduction, organs of, rudiments in, 189
Reptiles, longevity of, 50
Rhea, caeca of, 60, 77
Rhinoceros, longevity of, 54
Rhytina, 213
Riley, James, on food of Arabs, 174
Rimpau, on cultivation of rye, 326, 328
Rist and Khoury, on milk, 178
Rist, M., on ferment of Egyptian milk, 105
Rivière, M., on defecation in ostriches, 76, 78, 79
Robineau, Mde., 5, 6, 7, 8, 128, 159
"*Roman Elegies*," Goethe's, 268, 273
Rotifera, duration of life, 39
death of, 112
Roux, anti-syphilitic ointment, 146
Rovighi, on Kephir, 173
Rudimentary organs, 185 *et seq.*
Rye, duration of life of, 100
Rimpau's improvement of, 326
Salpétrière, hysterical patients at, 201
old women in the, 4, 5

Sand, M., on senile brain, 20
Sargent, on age of Sequoia, 98
Sauer-kraut, 165, 171
Sauvage, M., on atheroma, 30
Savage, on character of anthropoids, 193
Saxe-Weimar, Grand Duke of, and Goethe, 274
Schaudinn, spirillum of syphilis, 31
Schiller, Goethe on, 271
Schiller, on moral conduct, 310
Schlanstedt, rye of, 326
Schmidt, on microbes in constipation, 70
Schopenhauer, 235, 247, 255, 277, 330
Schumann, a degenerate, 134
Science, and morality, 301 *et seq.*
Sclerosis, in the aged, 31
Sea-anemones, longevity of, 47, 48
Sea-cow, 213
Selection, medical, 134
Seneca, 132, 235
Senescence, Brown-Séquard's specific against, 139
mechanism of, 25
phagocytosis as cause of, 35
Senility, characters of, 8, 14
and digestive system, 59
theories of causation of, 15 *et seq.*
Sensation, analysis of, with regard to pain and pleasure, 243
Sense of life, 26
of obstacles, 258
Sense, organs of, rudimentary structures in, 186, 187
"Sermon on the Mount," 321
Serums, cytotoxic, 147, 148, 149
Servants, care of, 321
Sex, and longevity, 57
Sexuality, Goethe and, 273 *et seq.*
and old age, 276
moral problems of, 305
Sexual organs, abnormalities of, 224
Sexual power and genius, 272
Shakespeare, quotations, 239, 307
Sheep, digestion of, 74
longevity, 55
Sight, rudimentary organs of, 189
Silos, 165
Siphonophora, 217
Skeleton, atrophy of, in the aged, 29
Sleep, and anæmia of brain, 122
and auto-intoxication, 120
and death compared, 125

Sleepiness, compared with hunger, 125
Sleeping-sickness, 124
Small-pox, and mortality rates, 144
Smell, analysis of, 243
Smell, rudimentary organs of sense of, 187
Smoking and longevity, 93
Social animals, 214, 220 et seq.
Socialism, 228, 229
Society v. the individual, 223 et seq.
Society, and morality, 306
Sociology, dependent on biology, 231
Sollier, Dr., on sensations at death, 130
Solomon, quotation from "Ecclesiastes," 233
Somnambulism, analysis of, 200 et seq.
Sorbose, fermentation of, 106
Soured milk, use of, 171, 181, 182
Sparrow, fecundity of, 58
Spencer, Herbert, criticism of Kant, 310
   criticism of socialism, 230
   theory of morality, 316, 322, 324, 327
Spermatozoa, in old age, 35
Spermine, 139, 140
Stadelmann, on lactic acid in diabetes, 170
Statistics on suicide, 3
Stature, in old age, 8, 9
Stein, Mde. von, 267, 268, 273
Steller's sea-cow, 213
Stern, M., on disinfection of intestine, 156
Stohmann, on digestion in sheep, 74
Stoics, 309
Stragesco, Dr., on digestion in mammals, 63
Strasburger, on disinfection of intestine, 156, 157
   on microbes in constipation, 70
Suicide, 3, 4, 237, 238, 265, 311
Sully-Prudhomme, definition of morality, 303
Suprarenal capsules, and atheroma, 32
Swimming, instinctive power of, 197, 198, 207
Syphilis, 31, 37, 145, 146, 302, 304
Switzerland, centenarians rare in, 91

Tanacol, as an intestinal antiseptic, 156
Taoism and immortality, 137, 138
Taste, analysis of, 243
Tavel, M., operations on large intestine, 152 et seq.
Taylor, Bayard, translation of *Faust*, 285
Termites, 220, 221
Testis, emulsion of, as used by Brown-Séquard, 139
   resistance of, to senescence, 35
Thanatology, 131
Theophrastus, 132
Thymol, as an intestinal antiseptic, 157
Thyroid, effects of extirpation of, 32, 33, 34
Timon of Athens, quotation from, 307
Tissier, Dr., on *Bacillus bifidus*, 161
   on use of lactic microbes, 181
Tissier, and Martelly, on putrid food, 164
Tobacco and longevity, 93
Tokarsky, on natural death, 126
Tolstoi, and death, 94
   "Death of Ivan Ilyitch," 318
Tortoise, 11, 12, 13, 51
Touch, sense of, in the blind, 257
Troubat, M., on instinctive swimming, 198
Trees, age and death of, 96, 97, 98
Trypanosoma, 124

Unicellular organisms, death of, 95
Urine, analysis of, in a centenarian, 7
Utilitarianism, 305

Vacherot, criticism of Kant, 313
Varenetz, 172
Vascular glands, relation to old age, 33, 34
Verworn, Max, on death in infusoria, 95
Vinegar, in preservation of food, 165
Vivisection, 301
Voisin, M., criticism of neuronophagy, 20
Voltaire, 92, 235
Volz, on swimming power of gibbons, 198

Wales, Mr., quotation from Riley, 174
Weber, Dr., on regimen for old age, 140, 141
Weichardt, on cause of fatigue, 122, 123

Weinberg, Dr., on preparation of human serums, 150
— on thyroid gland in aged, 33
Weiske, on digestion in sheep, 78
Weismann, A., on cause of old age, 15, 16
— on death in infusoria, 95
— on duration of life, 41, 43, 45, 51
"Weltschmerz," in German poetry, 236
Werther, Goethe's, 263, 267
Westergaard, statistics of mortality, 142, 144
Wiedersheim, on intestinal tract, 60
Wine, Goethe and, 271, 279
Wolff, J. H., Goethe's friend, 271
Women, education, 224 *et seq.*

YAHOURTH, use in intestinal putrefaction, 168, 170, 175, 177, 178
Yeast, conditions of growth, 106

ZEIGAN, Dr., on adrenaline, 122
Zell, Dr., on blind persons, 259
Zelter, Goethe's friend, 265
Zola, "La Joie de Vivre," 248
Zoological Gardens of London, 51, 81
Zortay, Pierre, age of, 87